EVERYTHING

YOU NEED TO KNOW ABOUT...

The
Menopause

EVERYTHING
YOU NEED TO KNOW ABOUT...
The
Menopause

DR RAMONA SLUPIK
WITH LORNA GENTRY

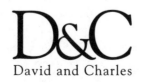

D&C
David and Charles

A DAVID & CHARLES BOOK
David & Charles is a subsidiary of F+W (UK) Ltd.,
an F+W Publications Inc. company

First published in the UK in 2005
First published in the USA by Adams Media, an F+W Publications Inc. company
as The Everything® Menopause Book in 2003

Project Manager Ian Kearey
Cover Design Ali Myer

A catalogue record for this book is available from the British Library.

ISBN 0 7153 2226 5

Printed in Great Britain by CPI Bath
for David & Charles
Brunel House   Newton Abbot   Devon

Visit our website at www.davidandcharles.co.uk

David & Charles books are available from all good bookshops;
alternatively you can contact our Orderline on (0)1626 334555 or write to us
at FREEPOST EX2110, David & Charles Direct, Newton Abbot, TQ12 4ZZ
(no stamp required UK mainland).

Everything You Need to Know About The Menopause is intended as a reference book only.
While author and publisher have made every attempt to offer accurate information
to the best of their knowledge and belief, it is presented without any guarantee.
The author and publisher therefore disclaim any liablility incurred
in connection with the information contained in this book.

Contents

Introduction

THE CHANCES ARE THAT IN THE YEARS APPROACHING YOUR OWN menopause, you have little time for (or interest in) reading up on the subject. You're busy, you're healthy and you're young! But the menopause isn't a condition confined to women who are retired, ill, old or unfit. Your body won't coordinate its menopause schedule with your appointment book, so you need to know something about the experience in order to be prepared for it. The menopause isn't a horrible condition or dramatic disease – it's an event, a passage, a personal evolution. Your job is to know how you can best care for your body during this time of transition.

So what is the menopause? How do you know when you're menopausal? What should you expect from the experience? And what can you do to manage your health through these important years of your life? That's what this book is all about.

There's so much information out there about the menopause these days – much of it conflicting or confusing – that it's easy to feel overwhelmed by it all. And every day new scientific developments change what we know about the menopause and the safety and effectiveness of common treatments. In this book you can find the best of the latest sound, proven information on the menopause, presented in simple, no-nonsense terms and an easy-to-use format. The book takes an in-depth look at the symptoms and stages of the menopause, options for managing your health through the experience, and important information about hormone replacement therapy and other treatment options. It offers some expert advice for dealing with common symptoms and side effects of menopause, and includes important ideas for maintaining a healthy diet and exercise plan to boost your overall physical and emotional fitness during the years preceding, during and following menopause. You can use it as a simple, accessible reference of vital information and helpful tips for making the most of your menopause.

And it's also worthwhile to talk a moment about... well, talking about the menopause. At some point, the menopause is a real event in every woman's life – an event that can have important repercussions for anyone who lives with and/or loves a menopausal woman. And although most women won't hesitate to discuss careers, children and other life issues with friends and family, many women find it difficult to talk about the menopause, fearing that it's too personal or socially unacceptable. This book doesn't encourage you to greet every stranger with a handshake and a hearty 'Well, I've been period-free for three months, how about you?' But it does teach some of the many ways that occasional talks with your friends and family about this important experience can be one of the first steps that can make your journey through the menopause more meaningful – and less stressful.

Remember, the menopause isn't an event defined by a chronological age, and it doesn't mean your life pauses or grinds to a halt. You can continue to enjoy the same quality of life after the menopause that you enjoyed when you were in your 40s – maybe even a *better* quality – if you look at the big picture and take some easy, preventative, good-health measures now. The road ahead can be fulfilling and rewarding if you're in the right frame of mind to enjoy it. Keep an open mind, take good care of your body, and explore your options.

CHAPTER 1

Every Woman's Menopause... and Yours

As women reach middle age, their world isn't neatly defined by their ageing reproductive functions. This chapter helps you explore all the changes that surround the menopausal experience to help you broaden your perspective of the challenges and opportunities offered by the menopause.

When the Menopause First Gets Your Attention

The menopause doesn't make a grand entrance – no fanfare, no bright lights, no day and date celebration of a definable event. The menopause becomes a reality for most women through a series of physical, mental and emotional changes – some subtle, some more dramatic – that tend to emerge, evolve, intensify and fade over a period of weeks, months and years. And the changes are unique to each individual, so women don't have a single 'menopause profile' to compare themselves to. The menopause can have many faces, and there's no one best way to prepare for or experience it. So how do you know when you are approaching the menopause?

Are You Anywhere in This Picture?

Consider the following. You're 40-something and life is pretty good. You've been at your current job long enough to feel that you have things under control (well, sort of). Your ideas and experience have earned you a fair amount of respect in your workplace, and every day you're a little clearer about who you are and where you want to go. Your family is maturing, too; with any luck, you spend less time chauffeuring, cooking and picking up after others, and more time gardening, working out at the gym, reading or maybe attending classes at a local community college. Your finances have been improving gradually over the years, and you may have a little more money now to indulge in the things you love best. And you're still young – you look ahead toward many long, happy years of health and well-being.

Of course, everything isn't perfect. Lately, for example, you've been having trouble sleeping – on some nights you can't fall asleep, while others find you waking in the middle of the night only to toss and turn your way back to sleep, maybe hours later. When the alarm goes off, you aren't really ready to get up and get going, because you haven't had much real, restorative sleep.

And you suppose the sleep disturbances are to blame for that occasional feeling of tiredness that overtakes you now and again. Some days, in fact, you just feel exhausted – you don't remember that happening much before, do you? And that exhaustion is probably to blame for your memory lapses. Stupid little things, really – sometimes you can't remember why you walked into a room, or what point you intended to make when you began speaking. Thank goodness you're too young to worry about Alzheimer's and senility (aren't you?)!

The UK has more people aged over 60 than under 16 for the first time, according to the 2001 national census. The census also revealed there were now 1.1 million people aged over 85 – a fivefold increase on the 1951 survey.

Even so, you find that you don't have much patience with friends and family who want to joke about your forgetfulness, do you? In fact, on some days you feel that you could easily snap the head off of the next person that says anything to you. In fact, it sometimes feels as if all your emotions are too close to the surface. Didn't you start crying over a stupid song on the radio when you were driving home last week? That's so unlike you!

But it's probably due to stress; you just need to take more time to relax. One look in the mirror can tell you that you're working yourself too hard, sleeping too little, or not eating and exercising properly. Even your skin looks tired, and your hair seems rather thin and limp. When did that happen?

And not to be too discouraging, but you seem to be putting on a little weight, too, which is totally unfair since you don't eat any more than you used to, and you're exercising more. Of course it's more difficult to resist those cravings for carbohydrates and chocolate all the time, but the weight gain you're experiencing seems well out of proportion to your occasional dietary relapses. What on earth is going on here?

Is This Perimenopause?

Now, the preceding example may not fit you to a T – you may be in your early 40s or even in your late 50s as you approach menopause. You may recognize only a few (maybe even none) of the symptoms listed in the example, while you seem to be experiencing several other symptoms that you don't remember experiencing before. But if any or all of this scenario seems familiar to you, what may be going on is called *perimenopause* – the time preceding menopause (the cessation of all menstrual periods) when associated endocrinological, biological and clinical changes occur. On average, women begin the perimenopause at 47 and experience it for about four years. But women can enter the perimenopause in their late 30s or early 50s, and it can last from a few months to eight or ten years. You have no way of knowing precisely when or how you'll begin noticing the changes that announce your coming menopause. Instead, you're more likely to find yourself one day connecting the dots of a number of odd symptoms and changes that eventually add up to the fact that you are, indeed, moving towards the menopause.

Whenever it happens, you're likely to have a difficult time accepting the idea that you actually are perimenopausal, but the realization can be a true relief. You may have decided that you were losing your mind or developing an odd and difficult-to-diagnose illness, when in reality, the symptoms you experience are normal, manageable demonstrations of a natural stage in your body's development.

To avoid unnecessary worry and discomfort about the menopause, don't deny the obvious. Learn all you can about what's happening to your body, and then take the necessary next steps to begin making your passage to the menopause as painless and productive as you possibly can. You've made a great start by picking up this book!

Just the Facts: What the Menopause Is and Isn't

The menopause is defined as 'The permanent cessation of menstruation resulting from the loss of ovarian follicular activity'. To put it simply, when you have your last period, you go through the menopause. Because your periods may become less regular and occur at greater intervals as you approach the menopause, however, you don't know you've gone through the menopause until 12 months have passed since your last period. So, by the time you know you've experienced natural menopause, you're already saying, 'Been there. Done that' to the whole menopause scene.

Natural versus Induced Menopause

You might have noticed that the preceding sentence mentions 'natural menopause'. Just as there's no one way to experience the menopause, there are multiple types of menopause, too:

- Natural menopause, described previously, is diagnosed when a woman has had 12 months of amenorrhoea (no periods) that is not the result of other physical or pathological conditions or treatments.
- Surgical or induced menopause occurs when a woman no longer menstruates as a result of having her ovaries surgically removed (with or without a total hysterectomy) or when ovaries stop functioning, either temporarily or permanently, as a result of chemotherapy, radiation, drug therapy or other medical treatments.

Note that having a hysterectomy doesn't mean you'll go through the menopause. If your uterus is removed but your ovaries remain, your body will continue to produce hormones. In this case, you don't experience the menopause as a result of your surgery, even though you won't have monthly menstrual bleeding.

Chemotherapy – the use of drugs to treat cancer – may not result in immediate menopause, but it can damage the ovaries. Depending upon the types of drugs your treatment involves, your ovaries might recover and function normally some time after treatment ends. In some cases, chemotherapy damages ovaries so severely that they cannot produce adequate amounts of hormones. In those cases, the menopause may occur months or even years after the therapy has ended. Doctors can't always predict whether damaged ovaries will recover.

Finally, pelvic radiation therapy can cause permanent ovarian failure (and therefore, premature menopause) when the ovaries are the target of high doses of radiation, for example, as treatment for cervical cancer. Since radiation therapy is a tightly targeted therapy, it often has no effect on ovarian function. If ovaries receive only low doses of radiation, they're likely to fully recover their functions.

Some estimates indicate that one in four women enters an induced or premature menopause. Because the onset of induced menopause is so abrupt, those women have no gradual adjustment period to prepare for postmenopausal changes. Women who have had both ovaries surgically removed, for example, may experience dramatic, abrupt menopausal symptoms, such as severe hot flushes or vaginal dryness.

If you face a premature menopause, make sure your doctor discusses all postmenopausal treatment options with you – including hormone replacement therapy.

What the Menopause Means

Whatever form of menopause you experience, the results are the same: you stop having periods, you stop being fertile, and you move into the post-childbearing phase of your life. That doesn't mean you become old as a result of menopause; according to the British Menopause Society (BMS), the average age of natural menopause in the Western world is 51. Most British women born after 1950 can expect to live until their mid-80s, meaning that the majority of menopausal women in the United Kingdom today have a half to a third of their lives to live after they've gone through the menopause.

But everyone's body is ageing all of the time. In the menopause, your body undergoes changes that require your attention. Your fluctuating hormones deplete your body's calcium, resulting in bone loss. As you age, you may become more susceptible to heart disease, diabetes and other illnesses. (Later chapters in this book discuss these changes and how you can best protect yourself from their negative consequences.) The menopause means you need to learn new ways to remain healthy, strong and vital.

But at the same time, the menopause also means that you have an opportunity to enjoy new levels of freedom and self-awareness. You may find that you don't miss the experience of menstruation at all. You no longer have to worry about becoming pregnant, so sex can take on new depths of pleasure. And the menopause is a marker of your evolving life; its arrival may encourage you to focus new attention and energy inwards, as you take this opportunity to evaluate who you are, what you're doing and where you want to go next.

What Causes the Menopause?

The average woman has about 400 reproductive cycles during her lifetime. In every cycle, the woman's pituitary gland produces follicle stimulating hormones (FSH) that trigger the follicle cells in the ovary that surround the developing eggs to produce oestrogen, which in turn prepares an egg (usually just one) for fertilization. As the body's level of oestrogen increases, the pituitary gland stops producing FSH and starts producing luteinizing hormone (LH), which causes the ovary to ovulate (release the egg) and produce progesterone, which prepares the uterine lining to accept the fertilized egg.

The mature egg is only one of several 'candidates' available each month. Those that don't mature (develop enough to be available for fertilization) are reabsorbed by the body. If the mature egg is unfertilized, it, too, is reabsorbed and the lining of the uterus is shed in the normal menstrual flow. The body's level of oestrogen dips, which then triggers the FSH production that starts the whole cycle again.

Every woman is born with a set number of eggs, ranging from 400,000 to 700,000. Half of those eggs deteriorate and are reabsorbed by each girl's body before she reaches puberty. Scientists are still researching why this occurs. With each month's ovulation, more of the egg supply is depleted. As you near menopause, your egg supply diminishes, your follicle cells stop responding to FSH and you stop ovulating. As a result – over a period of years – you stop menstruating and your ovaries stop making oestrogen and progesterone. You may continue to have menstrual periods after you stop ovulating, since your body continues to produce some oestrogen. Most women notice a change in the frequency, duration and flow of their periods during the three to four years before they stop menstruating completely. That's why you can't truly know that you've gone through menopause until a full 12 months have passed since your last period.

As the frequency of your ovulation decreases, the FSH levels in your bloodstream increase. In fact, your doctor can test the level of FSH in your blood to determine whether you're nearing menopause, which can be helpful if you're trying to determine your fertility.

What the Menopause Means for Your Hormones

Your body produces dozens of hormones, but only three of them play a major role in your reproductive cycle. Those three are oestrogen, progesterone and small quantities of androgens (testosterone, for example). Here's what those hormones do:

·   Oestrogen is a growth hormone that stimulates the development of adult sex organs during puberty; helps retain calcium in bones; regulates the balance of 'good' and 'bad' cholesterol in the bloodstream; and aids other body functions, such as blood glucose level, memory functions and emotional balance.
·   Progesterone balances the effects of oestrogen by aiding the maturation of body tissues and limiting their growth; stimulates the uterus, breasts and fallopian tubes to secrete nutrients necessary for the body to prepare for growing an embryo and bearing a child; and raises body temperature and blood glucose levels.
·   Androgens are male hormones produced in small quantities by the ovaries and adrenal glands – with the greatest quantities occurring at the midpoint of a woman's cycle – which contribute to a healthy libido by fostering a healthy desire for sex.

Many women incorrectly believe that their bodies stop producing oestrogen when they stop ovulating. As your body's supply of egg-producing follicles diminishes, the follicles that remain become less potent and produce lower amounts of oestrogen. In the perimenopause, cycles become less regular and some ovarian follicles don't mature to ovulation; when that happens, the body's level of progesterone drops.

When the pituitary gland senses that the ovaries aren't producing normal levels of hormones, it produces higher levels of FSH, trying to nudge the ovaries into producing more oestrogen. In the early stages of the perimenopause, that encouragement works; the follicles give up high doses of oestrogen, but the body still isn't producing the progesterone that normally rounds out the body's reproductive hormone mix. As a result, a woman in perimenopause may experience widely fluctuating levels of oestrogen for a number of years, until the ovaries shut down completely.

When oestrogen levels become so low that the lining of the uterus is unable to grow, menstruation stops. The body's FSH levels rise and remain high throughout the postmenopausal years. The body continues to produce small amounts of oestrogen, but in levels too small to support the hormone's age-defying functions in the body.

You Aren't the Only Thing That's Changing

Many women today enter their most productive years after the age of 40. Careers are established, children are growing older and more independent, a stronger sense of self emerges, and the pull of pop culture and social trends begins to fade in comparison to a growing inner strength and self-awareness. Although youth and beauty are often considered essential partners, many women are more beautiful at 40 than they've ever been before, a result of the increased economic and emotional stability and growing self-confidence that often accompany this period in life.

But most women of 40 are also approaching a decade of dramatic personal, physical and psychosocial change, a new stage of life that may be occurring at a time when they may be uninterested in – and maybe even resistant to – preparing for it. As personal as each woman's perimenopause may be, no woman is alone as she enters this phase of her life.

Britain Is Maturing

If you're in the perimenopause or have experienced the menopause, therefore, you're certainly not alone. Most perimenopausal and early postmenopausal women today are part of the 'Baby Boom' generation, the one born in the 1950s and 1960s. This generation is certainly among the largest and most influential of the current UK population, and they are among the first groups of women to have a new breadth of knowledge and information about the menopause experience.

Your Children Are Maturing

The other women of your age around the planet aren't your only companions in incredible change during these years. If you marry and have children in your mid to late 20s or early 30s, by the time you begin experiencing the first signs of perimenopause, it's quite likely that your children may be going through puberty and adolescence.

You went through puberty, so you know what your children are going through when they hit adolescence. Their bodies and minds are in turmoil. As children pass through relatively rapid physical changes (some they see as good, others horrify them), they also begin that important first round of 'Who am I?' introspection and exploration. They may feel confused, angry, loving, hateful, homeloving, childlike, adultlike, happy, depressed, bored, excited and lonely – and that's all just in the first 15 minutes after they wake up in the morning. If you think the dynamic of an adolescent's raging hormones can wreak havoc on a household, what about combining that loaded pistol with the fluctuating hormonal shifts of a perimenopausal mother?

When you and your child are both trying to work out who you are and what you want from life, even as you're trying to cope with changing physical and mental patterns in your life, the atmosphere is ripe for conflict. Of course, you also have a rare opportunity to connect with your child on a whole new level that women who aren't experiencing the perimenopause are unlikely to enjoy. But doing so requires a great deal of effort, patience and creativity on your part. You may or may not be able to turn this dual passage into a positive phase in your family's development, but you do have the opportunity to do so, and it's certainly worth the effort of trying.

Your Mate May Be Menopausal, Too

And what about your partner? You don't have to be in a same-sex relationship to experience 'couples menopause'. Although the phenomenon of male menopause was first the subject of research in the 1940s, even 20 years ago you would have had to search for scientific references to male menopause. Today, the medical and psychological communities treat the subject with much more respect.

You've probably heard the worn-out jokes about men going through a midlife crisis – a syndrome that somehow manifests itself in the male's acquisition of a wig or overuse of anti-grey-hair lotions, a 20-something trophy wife and a shiny red sports car. Well, many men do experience a psychosocial passage known as a midlife crisis, triggered by flagging sexuality, career plateaus and the realization that having it all isn't all it cracked up to be. But that midlife event, as important as it may be, isn't the same as male menopause.

Male menopause, known as *andropause* to the medical community, affects (by some reports) nearly 40 per cent of men between the ages of 40 and 60. All men begin producing less testosterone after the age of 40. As testosterone levels decrease, men may find that they experience fewer erections, that the erections are less easy to sustain, and that they experience longer intervals between erections. Male menopause can result in a wide range of symptoms in men, including lethargy, depression, mood swings, insomnia, hot flushes, irritability and decreased sexual desire.

Sexual dysfunction isn't the only marker of male menopause. Studies show that nearly 51 per cent of men aged 40 to 70 experience some level of impotence in varying degrees of severity and persistence – and that's many more than the number who exhibit symptoms of male menopause.

Diminishing testosterone in the bloodstream isn't the only culprit behind male menopause. Other factors include obesity, excess alcohol consumption, hypertension and the medications used to treat it, lack of exercise and other 'middle-age plagues' that damage health. While medications have been developed to treat erectile dysfunction, testosterone therapy is one of the few non-behavioural medical treatments available for combatting male menopause.

If you are in a same-sex relationship, the chances are very good that at some point you and your mate may both be experiencing symptoms of approaching the menopause. Although it may seem that sharing a household with another menopausal woman could lead to increased conflict, you also have a partner who may be better able to understand your experience. Both of you will need to remember, however, that every woman's menopause experience is unique, so neither of you can expect the other to have the same symptoms or reactions to those symptoms.

So what does this have to do with your passage through the perimenopause and menopause?

If you and your partner are both experiencing the mood swings, irritability and other negative effects of menopause at the same time, both of you may have a rougher time dealing with the experience. Your partner may or may not understand or accept his or her own struggle with midlife passage, and that could put extra demands on your patience and understanding – at a time when you won't feel particularly well-endowed with either. The essential message here is that your partner may not have the reserves of patience and support necessary to help you through all of the rough patches of the menopause, and at times you may have to draw on your deepest supply of those qualities to avoid throwing petrol on the smouldering fires of family discord.

And What about Your Ageing Parents?

And while you're surveying the vast horizon of family change that surrounds you during your perimenopausal years, don't forget about your parents. As you move into your 40s, 50s and 60s, your parents are pushing out ahead of you into the final stages of their lives. They're likely to be dealing with escalating health problems and diminishing self-reliance. You may find yourself called upon to help your parents make financial decisions, assist with the maintenance of their home, and lend other types of physical and emotional support.

Dealing with elderly parents can be demanding, and you may find these demands hitting you at a time when you're dealing with your own ageing process. Facing the realities of ageing in your parents can seem especially difficult when you're beginning to feel the effects of age. Expect some stress, and prepare yourself to deal with it.

Don't feel put off if other women in your family didn't (or don't) share your signs and symptoms. Every woman is unique in her perimenopausal experience – even within her own family.

Talking to Friends and Family

As you come up to 50, listen to what your friends and contemporaries who aren't experiencing the perimenopause say about it (on the rare occasion that the subject comes up). You're likely to hear comments similar to the following.

·   'I've made up my mind that I'm just not going to go through all those symptoms of the menopause; I'll fight it to the end!'
·   'I don't think it has to be such a dramatic thing; you just have to deal with it.'
·   'I'll be glad to go through it – I won't miss having periods, believe me.'
·   'My mum said she didn't even know she was in the menopause; her periods just stopped one day, and that was that.'

And those comments come from women. Men are more likely to comment on the subject only by making vague references to how much they dread having to deal with a woman in the menopause. Then they move on to another topic.

These comments and others like them used to lead anyone to believe that the menopause is all a state of mind. You could be strong and simply glide through the menopause without giving it the time of day, or you could fall on the sofa in a swoon and whimper for several years, until it was over. This old school of thought tells us that, like a fairy-tale monster that feeds on fear, the menopause exists only in the imagination and is best defeated by denying its existence. According to this philosophy, you won't have any problems with the perimenopause if you simply ignore it. It sounds great, but the perimenopause doesn't really work that way.

Communicate with People Who Matter

The information presented in the preceding sections tells quite a different story about what you may expect from the perimenopause. The perimenopause and menopause are real medical and psychological events, with some actual indicators and symptoms. The perimenopause is unique to each woman, so no one can know what you're feeling and experiencing during this time. You may experience no symptoms of the perimenopause, or you may have hot flushes or mood swings that you are certain everyone around you must notice. Bottling up your feelings and trying to hide your perimenopausal symptoms from your family or your close friends may seem like the best thing for them, but in fact, it's unlikely to help anyone – particularly you – understand and deal with the realities of this time in your life.

Though periodic mood swings, anger and irritability are common in the perimenopause, ongoing depression isn't. If your depression lasts more than a few weeks or if your family relationships seem to be on a non-stop downhill slide, talk to your doctor or community mental health service before the problem becomes unbearable.

One of the most important things you can do to make your perimenopausal experience sane and healthy (for you and your friends and family), is to communicate openly with them about your physical and emotional condition. Let your family and friends know what's going on with you. Talk about your symptoms and how they affect your mood, concentration, ability to sleep, level of anxiety or whatever applies to your experience. Answer their questions and ask for their understanding. If the perimenopause is making you irritable and impatient, try to establish some mutual rules for resolving family issues and avoiding unnecessary conflicts. Ask those you care about to help you find a way for everyone to move through the experience and emerge in one piece.

When It's a Family Affair

If you're sharing a life-changing moment with your child, you're going to have to be patient, strong and attentive. Your spouse or partner may have to step in and take a more active role in parenting, to relieve you of some of the stress and responsibility during certain phases of your perimenopausal changes. You may find that you need a mediator to work through some family difficulties – a relative, counsellor, teacher or family friend.

You and your partner may have to spend more time listening to each other and learning new patterns of behaviour. Things are evolving in your life, and therefore, in your relationship. Take this opportunity to revisit the way you think about your lover, life-mate, partner and friend and to begin interacting with that person on a deeper, more meaningful level.

You can rest assured that your mother and older female relatives have shared at least some portion of your experience in the perimenopause. As often as you've felt that you and your mother or other female relatives are from different planets, this is a stop you've all made on your life journey. You may find that this experience offers an opportunity to relate to your family in entirely new ways – and, with any luck, at least some of those ways will be positive!

Give Everyone a Break

Most importantly, try not to waste time judging yourself or your loved ones on the success rate of your communications and relationships during this time. If the perimenopause teaches anything, it is that you continue to be a work in progress. Later chapters in this book give you sound advice for making the perimenopause an easier, less stressful and more positive experience. But you can't expect every day to be a golden, glorious success.

Every day will offer new challenges and perhaps some new insights and opportunities to learn something new about yourself, your family, your colleagues and the ways you interact with all of them. If you give yourself a little room – accept the fact that once in a while you won't feel and act exactly as you may wish you could – you're more likely to give those around you a little more breathing room, too. Everybody's learning as they go; but when you enter the perimenopause, your body signals to you that your life lessons are about to become much more interesting.

CHAPTER 2

Understanding the Symptoms of the Perimenopause

Knowing what the perimenopause is doesn't really help you understand what it's all about. When you are aware of the range of symptoms that women have reported experiencing in the perimenopause, you gain a better understanding of the profile of common symptoms and know how to recognize those that masquerade as perimenopause, but may actually point to other issues in your physical and emotional health.

Taking a Closer Look at the Perimenopause

As stated, the perimenopause is the period of time preceding the menopause in which your body's reproductive system slowly winds down. Although the perimenopause differs for every woman, it generally marks a time of less-frequent ovulation and fluctuating levels of hormones, including oestrogen, progesterone and FSH. The perimenopause can last anywhere from two to ten years and usually begins sometime in a woman's mid- to late 40s. Eventually, your ovaries completely stop all egg production and menstruation permanently ceases – that's menopause.

But knowing when and why you stop menstruating doesn't help you prepare to take an active part in managing your health through the perimenopause and menopause. In fact, it's rather like being prepared for a trip to France with no more information than your airport names and flight times. Knowing that you fly out of Gatwick, spend an hour in the air, land at Charles de Gaulle airport, spend ten days in France, then return to Gatwick from Charles de Gaulle, doesn't do much to help you plan a good trip. And the average statistics of the menopause journey don't tell you much either. Although no one can describe exactly what your experience in the perimenopause and menopause will involve, some key bits of information about what others have experienced can help you prepare for the journey.

Consider this chapter your perimenopause orientation session. The goal of the information presented here is to help you feel more comfortable and relaxed when you experience the menopause, so you're better able to pass smoothly through every stop along the way, ready and able to deal with any problems you may encounter.

Don't let the term 'symptoms' lead you to believe that this chapter is describing the perimenopause as a disease or illness – it's neither. The perimenopause is a natural process of physical change. For the sake of simplicity, this book refers to the body's demonstrations of this natural process as 'symptoms', with no connotation of illness or disease.

Recognizing the Symptoms

So what can a woman expect from the perimenopause? What kinds of symptoms are common – or even possible – and what do they mean? If you have to listen to your body in order to understand its condition and needs, how do you interpret the messages of perimenopausal symptoms? And how do you know if your symptoms are related to the perimenopause or some other part of the ageing process?

First, it's important to understand that, if you think it may be the perimenopause, it probably is. No one is more familiar than you are with your body's feelings and reactions during your monthly cycles. As the following sections demonstrate, women have reported a wide variety of symptoms during and after the perimenopause. Remember, some women experience no symptoms at all.

It's also important to keep in mind that everyone can expect to experience some physical and mental signs of ageing. As women age, many of their physical changes are triggered or exacerbated by hormonal fluctuations. The good news is that any overt symptom that is associated with changing hormone levels can be temporary – and may even be diminished through diet, exercise or other therapeutic options. And above all, never forget that everyone's path to the menopause takes its own unique course.

What Women Experience in the Perimenopause

- 'I can't sleep at night; I wake up at two in the morning, worried sick about something that won't cause me a moment's concern at two in the afternoon.'
- 'My periods are spaced further and further apart, but other than that, I haven't had any special symptoms to speak of.'
- 'Do you think that when I wake up in the middle of the night feeling really warm, it could be a sign of something?'
- 'First, I'm screaming my head off at my husband, then I feel guilty and depressed about my behaviour. Is this the personality I'm going to have for the rest of my life?'

·   'I feel as if I gain ten pounds every time I look at a doughnut. I'm trying to exercise more and watch what I eat, but nothing I do seems to slow down my weight gain.'

Do any of those comments sound at all familiar? Couldn't some of them come from women at any age of their adulthood, or couldn't a few of them even have been made by a man?

The perimenopause isn't like measles; you don't wake up one day with a clear sign that you've come down with a case of waning oestrogen. So identifying when you enter the perimenopause isn't easy. If you start noticing obvious changes in the length of your periods, the intervals between them or the heaviness of your flow, and you're between the ages of 35 and 60, you should start checking for other signs of the perimenopause. But changes in your cycle may not be your first indicator that the perimenopause is approaching. Many women report symptoms of perimenopause while their periods remain much the same. Though we all have our own perimenopausal profile, most women feel some or all of the following symptoms as their bodies prepare to stop ovulating:

·   Hot flushes
·   Mood swings
·   Decreased sexual drive
·   Weight gain
·   Difficulty concentrating
·   Heart palpitations
·   Migraine headaches
·   Irregular and/or heavy periods
·   Involuntary urine release and bladder urgency
·   Insomnia
·   Vaginal dryness and painful intercourse
·   Panic attacks

Add to that list everything from aching joints and muscles to the onset of chin whiskers, and you've still only started to talk about the wide variety of symptoms that perimenopausal women have reported. Although some women report no symptoms of approaching menopause, more women do experience symptoms, so the chances are good that you will, too. Thinning hair, hot flushes, aching joints – these and other symptoms may seem like inevitable side effects of the ageing process. But many symptoms of the ageing processes can be triggered or exaggerated by the hormonal fluctuations of the perimenopause.

Staring Your Symptoms in the Eye

If the preceding list paints an ugly picture of the perimenopause, it's also important to mention here that even among women who experience one or more of these symptoms, their effects can be mild, transient or otherwise unannoying. Your body is adjusting to varying rates of hormones during the perimenopause; the signs and symptoms of that adjustment are often temporary, and disappear after your body has acclimatized itself to its new hormone levels. The following sections offer you a closer look at the causes of these symptoms so that you have a better idea of what to expect.

Don't dismiss symptoms or make up your mind that you're going to tough it out no matter what. You have options for alleviating symptoms – lifestyle changes, behaviour modification, hormone replacement therapy or dietary changes. Do yourself a favour and explore your options.

Hot Flushes (Including Night Sweats!)

Along with irregularities in menses, hot flushes have to earn the dubious honour of being one of the symptoms most commonly reported by women during the perimenopause. Nearly 75 per cent of women who report perimenopausal symptoms list hot flushes among them. Hot flushes can come at any time of the day or night, but when they occur during sleep, they're usually referred to as night sweats.

Not so long ago many doctors (predominantly men) considered hot flushes to be functions of the female imagination. Today, we know that hot flushes are real, physiological responses to the body's declining levels of oestrogen.

Hot flushes can be mild or severe, but in general, they involve a fast-spreading sensation of warmth in your neck, shoulders and face that may last a few seconds or as long as 30 minutes or more. This sensation may begin at the top of your scalp, behind your ears, on your chest or even across your nose. Hot flushes don't have to limit themselves to your head and shoulders; many women have also reported flushes occurring across the breasts, below the breasts or all over the body.

The flushes may be brief and cause only a slight flush on your face, neck or shoulders; by the time you notice them occurring, they're already beginning to fade. However, hot flushes can result in dramatic temperature rises that produce profuse perspiration on your upper lip, neck, forehead – or even your entire body. During a severe hot flush, the skin on your face, neck and scalp may become extremely red, and this flush may take longer to fade than the feeling of 'heat' itself. Some women have reported a rapid heart rate immediately before and during their hot flushes; some have experienced nausea and/or chills following hot flushes.

If you have hot flushes at night, they can contribute to sleeplessness, which can, in turn, contribute to anxiety, tension, mood swings or even depression. See Chapter 16 for ways to minimize the effects of hot flushes and accompanying night sweats.

Hot flushes may be accompanied by other feelings of physical discomfort, including tension, anxiety or nervousness. And, if you suffer hot flushes at night, in what most women call night sweats, you may experience some loss of sleep. Many women sleep right through their nighttime hot flushes, and know of them only when they awake in the morning to find their nightclothes or pillowcase slightly damp. Severe night sweats can produce such severe heat and sweating that sleep becomes impossible. Extended sleep loss can lead to feelings of anxiety, tension and even depression. But only a minority of women experience this severe form of hot flushes.

Irregular and/or Heavy Periods

Even if your periods have always been as regular as clockwork, you can expect some irregularities to occur in the years preceding the menopause. As you get older, you ovulate less frequently. The levels of oestrogen and progesterone produced in your body can flag and surge, contributing to unusually light or skipped periods, or periods that flow for weeks at a time. Some women experience spotting – or even phases of heavy bleeding – for a few days between periods. In other words, you may find that irregularity becomes the norm in your perimenopausal cycles.

What causes cycle irregularity during the perimenopause? Once again, the culprit behind the majority of heavy or irregular periods is hormonal fluctuations. In fact, hormone fluctuations can cause a variety of irregularities in your periods. As you enter the perimenopause, you might begin to ovulate less frequently. Because all hormone releases are triggered by others, an unusual fluctuation in one hormone can set off a series of unusual fluctuations in others, as your body tries to spur on or hold back the hormone in flux. For that reason, you might have a six-week cycle, followed by a four-week cycle, followed by a six-week cycle with unusually light flow, and so on. (A cycle is the length of time from the first day of one menstrual period to the first day of the next.) Your body is going through a series of starts and stalls as it attempts to adjust to fluctuating levels of hormones in your bloodstream.

Having said that heavy periods and ongoing irregular bleeding are not uncommon during the perimenopause, it's also important to have them checked by your health-care provider. Heavy bleeding or bleeding that continues for a long time can be more than an inconvenience. Non-stop heavy bleeding can leave you tired, weak and anaemic – a prime candidate for any cold, flu or infection you come in contact with. Even more importantly, heavy bleeding may have nothing to do with simple hormonal ebbs and flows. Between 30 per cent and 40 per cent of all women develop abnormal tissue in the uterus, such as fibroids or polyps, that begin to cause problematic bleeding during the perimenopause. Heavy bleeding could also be a sign of precancerous conditions or even endometrial cancer. Don't take chances that your period irregularities are just part of the change. If your irregularities are dramatic, see your doctor. (For complications of the uterus and their treatment, see Chapter 6.)

If periods come less than 21 days apart, last more than a week, are unusually heavy and maintain these irregularities for more than two cycles, make an appointment with your doctor or health-care professional for a gynaecological check-up.

Mood Swings

The good news about mood swings is that you may never experience them during the perimenopause. However, mood swings are a common complaint of perimenopausal women. Among women who cite symptoms in the perimenopause, nearly 50 per cent say mood swings are among the symptoms that bother them the most.

Whether you think of them as moodiness, temporary depression or simply the blues, mood swings can be minor 'speed bumps' in your day – or they can leave you feeling totally down and out. The experiences are as individual as the women who have them, but mood swings tend to take the form of intensified emotional reactions. Sometimes the swing can take you high, and you feel a particularly strong delight in everything around you – the weather, a film, your dinner companion. At other times, however, mood swings can take you on a wild roller-coaster ride of emotions, such as intense sorrow, despair, love, anger, anxiety, general depression or fear. A typical anger response during a mood swing can leave your heart pounding, your face flushed and your head throbbing. Mood swings can trigger bouts of crying and cause deep, dark feelings of hopelessness. Then, as nasty as they can be, mood swings may pass quickly, leaving you feeling shaken and confused by the emotional ride.

Although mood swings seem to be emotional responses, they can, in fact, be a direct physical response to the changing hormonal levels in your bloodstream. In fact, many perimenopausal women experience mood swings along with other common symptoms of premenstrual syndrome (PMS), even when those women have never before suffered from PMS symptoms. Those symptoms include a wide range of physical and emotional markers, including gastrointestinal distress, headaches, pains in muscles and joints, fatigue, heart pounding, hot flushes, exaggerated sensitivity to sounds and smells, agitation and insomnia.

Don't confuse mood swings with depression – feelings of despair, hopelessness, lack of energy and a diluted interest in life around you. When feelings of despair last more than a few weeks, you should consult your doctor. Untreated depression can damage your health and happiness.

Just as mood swings in the perimenopause can have both physical and emotional consequences, the causes of those mood swings can be both physical and emotional. First, consider that many of the symptoms of the perimenopause can cause emotional distress. Hot flushes can lead to sleeplessness, fatigue, irritability and anxiety. Those factors alone can make you feel angry, isolated and under siege – and contribute to occasional moodiness and transient depression.

Involuntary Urine Release

If you've ever experienced urinary tract infections (UTI), you may feel as though they're back with a vengeance during your transition into the menopause. And if you've never had urinary tract problems, you might develop them during the perimenopause. According to some estimates, nearly 20 per cent of all women over the age of 45 develop some urinary tract problems. Those problems can include UTIs, stress urinary incontinence (caused by a stressor such as sneezing, coughing or laughing) and urge incontinence (caused by a bladder spasm that forces urine out, even when the bladder is not completely full).

Many women are subject to UTIs on and off throughout their adult lives. But this problem can worsen during the perimenopause. Oestrogen contributes to the growth and nourishment of all cells and tissues. Because your body produces lower levels of oestrogen during the years leading to the menopause, the tissues lining the urinary tract can grow thin and more prone to bacterial infection and inflammation. That same lack of oestrogen-induced nourishment can weaken the muscles that surround your bladder and urethra. As a result, you experience more UTIs and other urinary tract disorders, a weaker bladder and less control over urine release.

Many urinary tract disorders have similar symptoms but require different treatments. If you suffer from burning or too frequent urination, involuntary urine release or a constant full bladder feeling, see your doctor for an accurate diagnosis and treatment.

As mentioned earlier, the most common kinds of urinary tract disorders that women experience during the perimenopause are stress urinary incontinence, urge incontinence and UTIs. These disorders can have similar symptoms, but they differ significantly.

Urinary tract infections are caused by bacteria in the urinary tract. The symptoms of UTI include feeling as though you need to urinate all the time, even when your bladder is empty; a burning sensation during urination; and – infrequently – small amounts of blood in your urine. Urinary tract infections can seem to fade, then return again. It's important to remember that, as with any bacterial infections, a full-blown UTI won't go away without antibiotic treatment. If left unchecked, the bacteria that cause a simple bladder infection can spread to the kidneys, causing a much more serious infection called pyelonephritis.

Urge incontinence is the result of a bladder spasm that forces urine out, even when the bladder is not completely full. These involuntary muscle contractions cause the bladder to release urine in varying amounts. Even though the woman may not feel as though her bladder is full and she needs to urinate, the sight, sound or even thought of water or urination can cause the sudden reflex need to urinate and an accompanying release of urine.

Stress urinary incontinence is another cause of periodic involuntary urine release. However, unlike urge incontinence that can result from the mere thought of emptying the bladder, stress incontinence usually has a specific triggering event, such as a sneeze or cough. Some women release small amounts of urine when they bend over, laugh or exercise.

Stress urinary incontinence is caused by weakened sphincter muscles, which surround the urethra, and can occur in women of any age. Women who have given birth, especially very large babies or difficult vaginal deliveries, often experience this disorder many years before they approach the menopause. But during the menopause, weakening sphincter muscles can contribute to the onset of stress urinary incontinence, even in women who have never experienced it. Obesity and chronic lung conditions that produce a lot of coughing, such as emphysema or cigarette smoking, can also cause or aggravate the condition. Certain strengthening exercises such as pelvic floor exercises, postmenopausal hormone therapy and even surgery are just some of the treatments used to combat this disorder. Losing weight and stopping smoking help, too.

A number of therapies can help end many urinary tract disorders. Biofeedback, pelvic floor muscle exercises and medication are just some treatment possibilities. Weight loss and bladder retraining can be successful tools in fighting incontinence, too. Have a talk with your doctor to find out more.

Changes in Libido

Few things are more individual than libido. Everyone has a unique attitude toward sex and sexuality, and certainly, we all differ in our sexual habits and desires. While this undeniable (and delightful!) individuality may seem to contradict any generalizations about how sexual desire can change during the menopause, many women do experience some types of changes during this time.

Many studies – including those of the famous Alfred Kinsey – indicate that both men and women can experience gradually declining sexual desire as they age. Pay special attention to the 'can' in that last sentence. It's important to remember that not everyone undergoes any noticeable change in libido during the menopause – in fact, many women don't. Still, many women in the perimenopause have reported noticeable changes in their level of sexual desire. Some say they have more interest in sex and enjoy it more, while others say their desires have diminished, and still others say they find sex increasingly unappealing – even painful. If the menopause is the trigger for this change, how can it differ so much between women?

To understand the answer to that question, remember that human sexuality is a complex and somewhat mysterious force, and changes in sexual desire are rarely explained by simple answers or attributed to single sources – no matter when those changes occur.

It's also important to remember that every woman's unique mind, body, relationships, attitudes and environment help to shape her sexual response. Her self-image and level of self-confidence play a supreme role. Understanding some of the physical and emotional factors that can affect libido during the perimenopause and menopause is an important first step in understanding your own sexual experience during this time of transition.

Hormones play a critical role in your body's sexual response. Oestrogen increases blood flow to all of your body's tissues, and it helps keep the walls of your vagina well-nourished and healthy. Oestrogen also helps maintain normal vaginal secretions and contributes to vaginal moistness and flexibility. As your body's hormone levels fluctuate through the perimenopause and then diminish after the menopause, you might experience some concurrent decline in sexual desire.

But that's not the whole story. Let's not forget those many women who report that their sex lives improve at this stage of life. The reasons for this not unusual phenomenon are relatively easy to understand. As women move into the perimenopause and menopause, they may have more access to quality time with a sexual partner. As children become more independent and then leave the family, interruptions and distractions diminish, allowing sex to be unhurried and spontaneous. After menopause, women can stop worrying about birth control, and therefore enjoy lovemaking free from pregnancy. And the growing self-confidence that comes with maturity can be a turn-on – to both the woman and her partner.

Weight Gain

The results are in: weight gain is commonly seen as people of both sexes age. And that isn't exactly new information. The term 'middle-aged spread' was coined decades ago to describe the tendency of the post-40 body to take on excess weight. Now, everyone doesn't gain weight during the perimenopause and after the menopause, and not everyone who does gain weight gains debilitating amounts. But, the fact is that the majority of women report weight gain at this time. Even women who don't gain weight may experience a change in their body shape. Many women in middle age gain softer, rounder abdomens, larger hips, thicker waistlines and even extra weight on their shoulders, arms and thighs.

Your body's metabolism changes as you move into middle age. As you age, your body burns calories much more slowly (some studies say by as much as 4 to 5 per cent) as each decade passes. So, instead of burning off the calories that you eat, your body converts them into fat. You may feel as though you aren't eating any more, and may actually feel you are eating less, but your body's furnace just needs less fuel to perform the same functions.

Although you may feel as though you are always on your feet and very active, many people slow down a bit as they move into middle age – running fewer errands, doing less physical work around the house and so on. All of these factors contribute to unwanted – and sometimes unhealthy – weight gain during the perimenopause and after menopause.

Difficulty Concentrating

If you're approaching 50 and it seems as though you aren't quite as sharp mentally as you used to be, it's probably because you aren't. Although fuzzy thinking, forgetfulness, difficulty concentrating and memory problems are common complaints of perimenopausal and menopausal women, these issues are linked as closely with the ageing process as they are to changing ovarian functions. Today, doctors and health-care professionals recognize that certain cognitive problems are due to depleted oestrogen levels and other changes in the ageing brain.

Can oestrogen supplements help women in the perimenopause think more clearly?
Some of the brain's midlife slowdown results from loss of healthy neurons. Some studies have shown that oestrogen can help heal damaged neurons and increase other neurotransmitters that govern memory and other mental functions, but other studies haven't supported these results. Studies continue, so watch for developments.

How does this fuzzy thinking manifest itself? In ways you've probably experienced most of your life – for example, losing your car keys, forgetting what you were about to say, recognizing a face but failing to recall the name, searching fruitlessly for the right word, being easily distracted or losing your train of thought. As women reach the age of menopause (around 50), however, they can suffer an increase in these sorts of problems. You may have heard people refer to these lapses as 'senior moments', and if you're approaching the age of menopause you're likely to be experiencing them yourself. The ageing process affects the brain, as it does in all the other parts of the body.

While you can't stop your brain's odometer from registering the passing years, you can slow down and repair many of the issues that contribute to fuzzy thinking and other cognitive roadblocks. See Chapter 19 for more information.

Heart Palpitations

Heart palpitations are the sudden uncomfortable awareness that your heart is pounding, often at a more rapid rate than normal. Heart palpitations can be frightening, but remember that they aren't uncommon in perimenopausal and menopausal women. Certainly these women aren't the only ones to experience palpitations – many men and women have them after exercising, when frightened or while taking some medications. But at the menopause, the instances of heart palpitations seem to rise in women. Their frequency and severity vary from woman to woman, but under normal circumstances they aren't a problem. If they get out of hand, however, occurring in rapid succession, heart palpitations can cause problems.

Women describe heart palpitations differently, but in general a heart palpitation feels like your heart is beating rapidly, out of sequence, too strenuously or in some other abnormal fashion. A heart palpitation can feel like no more than a brief fluttering in your chest that passes within a matter of a few seconds. Other, stronger palpitations can feel like a distinct pounding in your chest that lasts a few minutes and can leave you feeling light-headed or short of breath.

If your heart palpitations are severe or produce significant discomfort or side effects, you need to talk to your doctor or health-care provider about them. Some palpitations are a warning sign of an impending heart attack. Pay attention to the number and frequency of your palpitations, and be prepared to discuss these and your heart history when you talk to your doctor.

Heart palpitations can be caused by anxiety or some other system-stimulating problem, such as too much caffeine or an overactive thyroid gland. Blood glucose levels that are either too high or too low can also contribute to heart palpitations. Palpitations that are present on waking are particularly worrisome. As you move into the perimenopause, your body's fluctuating hormone levels can contribute to all of these causes. The good news about this symptom is that heart palpitations associated with the perimenopause and menopause tend to run their course and stop after the body adjusts to postmenopausal hormone levels.

Caffeine, cigarettes and excess sugar can overstimulate your system and be a contributing factor in heart palpitations. The perimenopause is a great time to cut back on your intake of these.

Migraine and Other Headaches

Technically, migraine headaches aren't considered a symptom of menopause. Nevertheless, many women who have never experienced a migraine in their lives begin having them during the perimenopause. These hormonally related migraines are often experienced by younger women in the few days before their periods. In both cases, fluctuations in your body's oestrogen levels seem to be a cause.

Although both sexes suffer from migraines, women are three times more likely to have them. Migraines are intensely painful headaches thought to be associated with constricted blood vessels in the brain. Women who suffer migraines describe them as pounding headaches that can cause nausea, vomiting and a strong sensitivity to light, noise and odours. Some migraine sufferers – almost a third, according to some studies – report a certain premonition, or aura, for several minutes before the actual pain begins. This aura can include flashing lights, certain odours, changes in their vision or numbness in a hand, arm or leg. Migraines usually last four or more hours, and they can last as long as a week.

Migraines aren't the only kind of headaches that seem to accompany the perimenopause. In general, women report having more frequent and severe headaches during this time. These are usually simple stress or muscle tension headaches, and are often relieved by over-the-counter analgesics such as aspirin, ibuprofen and paracetamol.

Insomnia

Interruptions in normal sleep patterns are common complaints of perimenopausal and postmenopausal women. During the years approaching the menopause, many women find that they wake once or twice during the night and then have a difficult time returning to sleep. Other times, women find that it takes longer for them to fall asleep when they go to bed at night, or that they awaken an hour or two earlier than they used to. Whatever form it takes, insomnia leaves women feeling tired, irritable and out of touch with their surroundings.

This chapter has already discussed many other conditions of the perimenopause that logically contribute to sleeplessness – night sweats, anxiety and the need for frequent urination. But the root causes of insomnia during these transitional years go even deeper. As we age, most people establish new sleep patterns. Although some women go through a phase during the perimenopause in which they actually require much more sleep than they have previously, others experience periods of wakefulness and restlessness during hours that they previously would have been deeply asleep. Stress, changes in diet, the need for frequent urination, heartburn, hot flushes and anxiety are a few of the different factors that can trigger insomnia. And the factors that prevent you from falling asleep when you first go to bed at night can be very different from those that wake you and keep you awake in the middle of the night.

tips

Most health-care professionals agree that certain lifestyle habits can contribute to insomnia – at any time in your life. Take regular exercise and try not to consume any alcohol, sugar, caffeine or rich foods within the two to three hours before bedtime.

Fortunately, many women find that insomnia is a transient problem that may last no more than a few months. For others, insomnia during the perimenopause may be so severe that it hampers their performance and sense of well-being during the day. Chapter 10, 'Your Mind, Mood and Emotional Health', offers a number of good options for minimizing insomnia when it strikes. As always, if your symptoms become severe, consult your doctor or health-care professional. You can combat insomnia, so don't allow it to drag you down during this important transition phase.

Stay on Top of Your Symptoms

As you have seen in this chapter, a wide range of symptoms can appear during the years preceding the menopause. But it's important to remember that, as noted at the beginning of this chapter, you may experience none, some or all of these symptoms – or others that aren't even listed. To be certain that you are doing all you can to maintain peak health during this important time of transition, pay close attention to your body and don't ignore the messages it sends you. Many of the symptoms that initially seem par for the course for middle age may be symptoms of problems requiring serious and quick medical treatment. So don't ignore any ongoing problem because you think it's just the change. Work closely with your doctor to make sure that your body gets any and all the help that it needs to stay strong, fit and healthy.

CHAPTER 3

Passing Through the Stages

Since women of 50 today may have more than a third of their lives ahead of them, it's important that they understand the changes their bodies are experiencing. Tracking the progress of your own journey towards and through the menopause will help you feel more comfortable and secure about where you are – and ready to enjoy the years ahead.

A Traveller's Guide to the Menopause

When we talk about the stages of perimenopause and menopause, we're really talking about the normal ageing process – a subject that's become nearly taboo in our youth-oriented Western culture. Fortunately for our burgeoning post-50 population, however, ageing today is a happier, healthier business than it was even 30 years ago. We're living longer, healthier lives now. Medical advancements have made the age of 50 more of a midway marker than the opening of the final scene that it used to be. Remember, the menopause isn't really something you go through, although that's often the easiest way to describe the period of change that most women experience in the years preceding and following full, natural menopause. The menopause is merely one event in the long journey women make as they move away from their reproductive years and into their post-reproductive years.

This transformation takes place in stages that occur, for most women, over a period of decades. Although every woman's body chemistry and, therefore, age experience is unique, many experts agree that most women typically experience the following physical changes on the menopause journey, however.

- **Perimenopause** – the years when a woman's oestrogen production gradually decreases as a natural result of ageing – typically occurring during a woman's mid-40s.
- **Menopause** – the time when ovulation ceases and oestrogen production falls to such low levels that all menstruation stops for at least 12 months in the case of natural menopause, or immediately in the case of surgical or induced menopause. Many women enter natural menopause in their 50s.
- **Postmenopause** – the years following the menopause.

The following sections detail each of these stages. But to put the changes that occur in the perimenopause in perspective, take a moment to review the starting point from which most women embark on the journey towards the menopause.

The term 'premenopause' is no longer used to refer to the years preceding the menopause, because all the years of a woman's life that precede the menopause are premenopause. Today, 'the perimenopause' is used to describe the years when a woman's reproductive system slows down as it approaches the menopause.

The Phases of Menstruation

Women in their teens, 20s and early 30s who have typical reproductive functions experience monthly menstrual cycles. Some people label these years as 'the reproductive years', but it's important to remember that as long as you ovulate and have periods, you are fertile and you can conceive. For the purposes of this book, therefore, it is helpful to think of this life stage as that of your early adulthood, which lasts, for the average woman, into her 40s.

By the time most women reach their late teens, they ovulate regularly, and their bodies establish their 'normal' reproductive cycle. Although the length and regularity of the cycle varies from woman to woman, you can think of the typical reproductive cycle as occurring in two main phases:

· **Build-up (follicular phase):** the time when one of the ovaries begins developing an egg for release, starting on the first day of menstrual bleeding and continuing until midway through the cycle when ovulation occurs.
· **Premenstrual (secretory phase):** the time following ovulation when the uterine lining develops in preparation for nourishing a potential fertilized egg.

Hormones trigger each event that occurs during the two phases of one complete menstrual cycle. Here's a rough overview of what happens:

1. On Day 1 of the menstrual cycle, the body begins to shed its built-up uterine lining and the pituitary gland releases follicle-stimulating hormones (FSH) to prompt the ovaries to produce oestrogen in order

to prepare an egg for ovulation, which develops in one follicle in one ovary. (Occasionally more than one egg matures in the same cycle.)

2. FSH levels pulse occasionally through the next 13 days as oestrogen levels gently rise to their peak.

3. On around Day 14, the pituitary gland releases luteinizing hormone (LH) to make the ovary release the egg and to turn the follicle cells that surrounded the egg into a progesterone-producing machine.

4. For the next two weeks or so, oestrogen production slowly diminishes as progesterone production steps up, and the two hormones work together to spur the lining of the uterus to thicken in preparation for accepting and nourishing the fertilized egg.

5. Towards the end of the cycle (around Day 28), the egg reaches the uterus. If fertilized, the egg embeds in the lining and oestrogen and progesterone levels remain strong. If the egg is unfertilized, all hormones – FSH, LH, oestrogen and progesterone – drop to minimum levels and the lining of the uterus begins to fall away as menstrual flow, which takes us back to Day 1 of the cycle.

According to some studies, your menstrual cycles may shorten before the age of 40, then lengthen slightly as you approach the menopause. So, while your period may occur every 26 days when you're 40 years old, as you reach 45, 35-day cycles may be normal for you.

This cycle may take 21 days in some women or as many as 35 days in others. Studies have shown that your age may play a critical role in the length of your menstrual cycle. If your cycles fall outside this range, you should discuss this with your doctor.

Fast Facts about Premenstrual Syndrome

Even when you've established your own individual cycle and are in the height of your reproductive years – from your late 20s to your mid-30s –

your monthly cycle may not proceed as a smooth ride. Most women experience some symptoms associated with their menstrual periods, including cramp, swollen and tender breasts, mood shifts and headaches. These symptoms can also be present – in addition to others – in premenstrual syndrome (PMS). Some research indicates that PMS can include as many as 150 separate symptoms, but all symptoms of PMS fall into two major categories:

- Physical symptoms of PMS include bloating, water retention, pelvic pressure or cramp, and headaches or migraines.
- Emotional symptoms can consist of irritability, mood swings, difficulty concentrating and food cravings.

Some women never have PMS, while others – some studies estimate a third of all women – may have episodes of it throughout their adult lives. These women often find that PMS is most frequent and severe during their 30s. Many women who have never experienced PMS or have had only occasional, minor symptoms, report severe PMS phases as they enter the perimenopause.

Although PMS symptoms can occur anywhere from midway through your cycle to a few days after you begin your period, no one symptom should ever last more than two weeks. If you have any symptom longer than 14 days, report it to your doctor.

A less common, but even more debilitating, type of premenstrual syndrome is premenstrual dysphoric disorder (PMDD). Women who suffer from PMDD often experience severe depression, anxiety, sleep disturbances and fatigue in addition to a wide range of physical disturbances. Although these two syndromes differ in severity, diagnosis and treatment, both seem to be linked to the way the body processes and responds to reproductive hormones. (See Chapter 11 for more information.)

Doctors diagnose PMS and PMDD based on when a woman's symptoms occur, not just the symptoms themselves. If you want to check your own premenstrual symptoms, you can keep a menstrual journal. If symptoms are repeated at specific intervals, they may indicate PMS.

The Journey Through the Perimenopause

During the perimenopause you may experience the classic symptoms discussed in Chapter 2, including irregular and/or heavy periods, mood swings, hot flushes, weight gain and headaches.

Alternatively, you may experience increased severity of PMS symptoms. PMS and some symptoms of the perimenopause mirror each other because both are thought to be caused by fluctuating levels of reproductive hormones. Some women are more sensitive to these fluctuations than others, which explains why some women have no symptoms and others have symptoms that are severe.

Don't read too much into new and more severe PMS symptoms. Although they can signal that your reproductive system is slowing down – and that means that you're moving into the perimenopause – they can also signal a new awareness of your body, or your body's reaction to the increasing stresses of life.

Chronicle Your Symptoms

But how do you know whether or not you're truly experiencing the perimenopause? Your doctor or health-care professional can help to determine that with tests discussed later in this chapter. But remember – most diagnoses of the perimenopause aren't based on symptoms so much as on when symptoms occur. So if you have begun to notice changes in your monthly cycle or other symptoms associated with the perimenopause, you can begin the diagnostic process yourself by keeping a menstrual calendar.

You can use any system that works for you, but here's an example of how the menopause calendar can work. Perhaps you have been experiencing periodic waves of anxiety and depression, along with bad headaches and occasional hot flushes. And occasionally your craving for sweets and carbohydrates gets totally out of control. You can use a menopause calendar to track those symptoms, to see if they're associated with specific days of your monthly cycle.

To begin, you need a simple calendar – you can use a desktop calendar, appointment book, wall calendar, electronic calendar file, journal or any medium you like, so long as your calendar lists days and dates and provides room for you to record your daily notes. To save room, devise some abbreviations for symptoms and events, such as:

H	Headache
An	Feeling anxious
CC/SC	Carbohydrate cravings/sweet cravings
D	Depressed
HF	Hot Flush
P	Period (menstrual)
GM	General mood

Finally, you need to have a rating system to rank the severity of your symptoms. That way, if you have a mild headache one day and a migraine on another, you can check the difference. Similarly, you can note how light or heavy your flow was on any day of your period. You may choose to rank severity with a scale of 1 to 5, with 1 being least severe/lightest and 5 being most severe/heaviest. You can use this ranking to note your general mood, too, with 5 meaning 'feeling horrible' and 1 indicating that you're feeling great. Add new symptoms as they occur, so you can get a full picture of how your health and how you feel changes from day to day. Don't be compulsive about your calendar, but make sure it notes cyclical symptoms and menstrual dates. Some doctors or health-care providers might even offer you their own standard version of a symptom calendar, such as the one shown in FIGURE 3-1.

FIGURE 3-1: MENSTRUAL SYMPTOM DIARY

You can begin recording your symptoms on any day you choose, though some like to start on the first day of their period. Here's one example of a menstrual symptom calendar.

Name:

Weight (cycle day 1):

Severity of symptoms:

☐ None ◪ Moderate

⊟ Mild ■ Severe

Cycle day	1	2	3	4	5	6	7	8	9	10	11	12	13	14	15	16	17	18	19	20	21	22	23	24	25	26	27	28	29	30	31	32	33	34	35
Date																																			
Menses																																			
Nervous tension																																			
Mood swings																																			
Irritability																																			
Anxiety																																			
Depression																																			
Forgetfulness																																			
Crying																																			
Confusion																																			
Insomnia																																			
Weight change*																																			
Swelling of extremities																																			
Breast tenderness																																			
Abdominal bloating																																			
Headache																																			
Craving for sweets																																			
Increased appetite																																			
Heart pounding																																			
Fatigue																																			
Dizziness or faintness																																			

*Please record the difference between today's weight and the weight on cycle day one. For example, if you weighed 63kg on the first day of your period and now you weigh 65, enter +2; or if you weigh 66, enter +3.

Every day note on your calendar any symptoms you experience and their severity ranking. Note the first and last days of your period, and how light or heavy your bleeding is each day. Keep the calendar for at least three months to get a good roadmap of recurring symptoms and your cycle's regularity or irregularity. This information can help you – and your doctor – spot symptoms that might be associated with the perimenopause.

Many women have found that simply tracking and understanding the cyclical nature of their perimenopausal symptoms makes those symptoms less severe and intrusive. For example, if on the 21st day of your cycle every month you're prone to feeling anxious or depressed, but that the feeling passes by Day 23, those feelings may seem less severe and debilitating. If you expect to develop a sore throat sometime within the second week of your cycle, you aren't worried by its appearance every month. Don't misunderstand this message – keeping a menstrual calendar won't cure your perimenopause symptoms. But information is power: the more you know, the better able you are to make strong, informed decisions about how to respond to your symptoms.

If you have a sudden onset of extreme symptoms – such as severe headaches or extremely heavy bleeding – that lasts more than a few days, see your doctor. Severe long-lasting symptoms may be related to some serious illness or disease, and you should report them straight away.

If You Need to Talk to Your Doctor

When your symptoms of perimenopause cause too much disruption in your life, it's time to talk to your doctor. Health-care providers can help to determine whether or not the perimenopause and its accompanying hormonal shifts are contributing to the symptoms you're experiencing, and how you best can treat them. Doctors can test for conditions of the perimenopause by checking hormone levels in your blood. (Newer saliva tests are currently being developed, but most medical experts don't yet consider them reliable.) Those tests may check for levels of oestrogen, FSH and LH – your doctor determines which hormones to check, based on your symptoms and health history. Rising levels of FSH, for example, can indicate that the body is ovulating less frequently and FSH is being released from the pituitary gland in greater quantities to help spur on the ovaries' production of oestrogen. Many doctors consider an FSH level of 40 or above to be a firm indicator that the menopause has occurred. FSH levels can fluctuate in the perimenopause, so sometimes a single test doesn't provide enough information on which to base a diagnosis.

The point of keeping your menstrual and PMS symptom calendar is to show it to your doctor, so remember to take it with you to your appointment. Some hormone testing may be best performed on certain days, and your doctor will need the information you've recorded to determine when to schedule your test.

If your doctor diagnoses you as being perimenopausal, he or she will talk to you about possible treatment options. Chapter 11, 'Understanding Hormones and HRT', and Chapter 12, 'Alternatives to Hormone Replacement Therapy', give more information on these topics. Remember, your symptoms may go through a number of changes or even resolve themselves with no treatment at all. In fact, some estimates say that as many as 55 per cent of women in the perimenopause use no treatment of any kind. In many cases, your body slowly adjusts to its changing hormone levels and your symptoms remain mild or even unnoticeable. (Unfortunately, most women whose menopause is artificially induced have more pronounced, severe symptoms, and are more apt to require hormone replacement therapy or other treatment options.)

If you're in the perimenopause you have a number of options, and your doctor can help you explore all of them. It's important that you have a doctor who you feel completely comfortable with at this important time. Chapter 5, 'Working with Your Doctor', discusses that relationship.

Other Physical Changes During the Perimenopause

Recognizing the unique experience each of us has as we age, most of us can expect to experience other physical changes during – and perhaps as a result of – the physical changes of the perimenopause. If the perimenopause occurs during a woman's 40s, for example, here are some of the changes her body might be undergoing:

·   Muscles may lose mass easier and become harder to tone during your 40s, so your old exercise plan may not be enough to maintain the strength and body weight you enjoyed in your 30s. You may need a new exercise programme during this time; see Chapter 14.

·   Bones can start to lose calcium as oestrogen levels recede and the body becomes less efficient at absorbing calcium from food. You may need to adjust your diet to include more vitamin D and calcium, or consider taking supplements. See Chapter 8 for more information.

·   Eyes become less efficient as the lenses lose elasticity and their controlling muscles weaken, making focusing close-up more difficult. Oestrogen helps keep eyes and muscles elastic, so diminishing levels of oestrogen contribute to this degeneration.

·   Skin and hair can begin to thin in response to lowered levels of oestrogen; most people start to get some grey hair in their 40s. Oestrogen also helps maintain the collagen content (the basic protein bridgework) of your skin, thus keeping it youthful and elastic. Your strong ally in the battle against this ageing factor is a healthy diet and lots and lots of water. See Chapter 15 for more information.

·   Metabolism slows down during your 40s, so weight gain can creep up on you, even if you maintain your previous diet and exercise plan. Typical dieting methods are unlikely to work as well for you at this age, so maintaining or losing weight may require additional exercise and calorie-cutting.

·   Propensities for certain conditions, such as diabetes and asthma, can accelerate during this time, due to changing hormone levels, lowered resistance to stress and infections, and other factors of ageing. Medical check-ups and health maintenance are more essential than ever at this point; see Chapter 6.

Don't be put off by this list; yes, the ageing process does involve physical changes and even some deterioration of your body's systems. But there's never been a time when medicine and health care, public information and healthy life practices have been better able to contribute to everyone's pursuit of a healthy, active middle age. You have more control than any generation that's preceded you in how quickly or slowly your body loses ground to the ageing process. You can learn ways to manage the effects of the perimenopause and its role in the ageing process.

If you've been casual about your health until you hit 40 (which most of us are), now is the time to get serious about preparing for a long, healthy life ahead. Diet, exercise, lifestyle changes and regular medical check-ups are your strongest agents for maintaining a strong, healthy body.

The Menopause and the Years Ahead

If you still have both of your ovaries as you move into your 50s, the chances are good that you'll stop having menstrual periods altogether. When you've not had a period for 12 months, it's official – you've experienced natural menopause. So you stop having periods – but what other changes take place as a result of this transition? And what lies ahead?

Hormones Take a Dive after the Menopause

After the menopause, oestrogen and progesterone levels plummet. Although other parts of your body continue to produce some hormones, they cannot compensate fully for the loss of ovarian hormone production. The specific role of these hormones is treated in Chapter 11, but some of the major postmenopausal side effects are increased bone loss and the drying and shrinking of the vagina (vaginal atrophy). Fewer vaginal secretions are produced when there is no oestrogen, so your vaginal wall becomes less lubricated and flexible and more prone to tears and cracking. In fact, all of your skin tissue becomes thinner and less elastic, including the muscles that surround your urethra (the opening to the bladder). That's how diminishing hormone levels can contribute to involuntary urine release through stress incontinence.

Your cardiovascular system misses those hormones, too, with their beneficial impact on HDL cholesterol and their inhibiting effect on LDL cholesterol. And just as your arteries become more susceptible to plaque build-up, they begin to narrow and lose elasticity. As a result, oestrogen loss can contribute to heart disease.

Another important side effect of plummeting hormones is a rapid advance of the bone loss that began in your 40s. In the first five years that follow the menopause, women can lose as much as a quarter of their bone density – a potentially deadly development. Bone fractures that develop as a result of osteoporosis can have life-threatening consequences. This bone loss slows down for most women within a decade or so of the menopause, but without supplements or HRT, it continues throughout a woman's life.

Hot flushes can continue for a period of years after the menopause, but in most cases, diminish entirely within five years. See Chapter 16, 'Coping with Hot Flushes', for ways to minimize the effects of hot flushes.

Other Postmenopausal Changes

During your 50s and early 60s – the decades immediately following the menopause – your body undergoes some inevitable changes resulting from the natural ageing process. Again, your body is unique, and so are your family medical history, your lifestyle and your individual health programme. But in general, here are the types of changes many women experience in the years that follow the menopause:

·   Hearing loss can set in, due to the ear canal tissue's becoming thinner and drier. Many people have no hearing loss until they are in their 60s, but almost a third of women over 65 report hearing problems. You can keep this loss to a minimum by protecting your ears from loud noises. Wear earplugs when you mow the lawn and avoid sitting close to loud stereos and televisions. And have annual hearing check-ups, so you know when your hearing loss reaches the you-need-a-hearing-aid stage.

- Joints lose cartilage with age, and connective tissue becomes less flexible and resilient, making arthritis and other types of joint pain more common in ageing women. Exercise and weight control are critical factors in maintaining healthy joints.
- Lungs become less elastic as we hit our mid-50s, which can contribute to shallower breathing and, therefore, less oxygen in our bloodstream. Get plenty of aerobic exercise to keep your lungs pumping. And, if you're still smoking, stop now!
- The brain loses mass and shrinks slightly with each passing year. As a result, women can face impaired cognitive functions as early as 70. Keep your body and mind active – participate in a regular aerobic exercise programme, do crossword puzzles, learn to use a computer, visit family and friends, read the newspaper and travel. Life's pleasures are also your best weapon in keeping your mind alert and agile. Remember, if you use it, you don't lose it.
- Digestion slows down as we reach our 60s, and food moves at a slower pace through our intestines. As a result, many postmenopausal women report problems with constipation. Eat plenty of whole grains, fresh fruit and vegetables, and drink plenty of water to combat this change in your digestive function (and, you guessed it, exercise).

Living for the Rest of Your Life

These changes contribute to the challenges you face in maintaining your strength and health as you move through the postmenopausal years of your life. Although ageing is inevitable, you exercise tremendous control over its effects. The menopause demands that you pay attention to your body, make decisions and take actions that can protect and nurture it through the many years ahead. But the menopause also can usher in a time of great freedom, personal exploration and growth. How you manage the symptoms of the perimenopause and the realities of ageing that follow will determine your own postmenopausal experience. The remaining chapters of this book take a closer look at all the health issues that surround the menopause, and offer simple, effective and smart ideas for managing your health and combatting these issues – now and for the rest of your life.

CHAPTER 4

Why Your Attitude Matters

As you approach the menopause, you may not have evaluated your attitude toward the transition you are making. The way you think about the menopause, ageing, change and your own self-worth is all-important at this time of physical and emotional transition. This chapter offers you some key techniques for assessing just how you feel about the menopause – what hopes and fears you bring with you to the perimenopause and the menopause.

Is It Time to Check Your Attitude?

Women approaching the menopause today have much to be thankful for. At no previous time in history have we known more about both the biology and psychology of the menopause and ageing. We've never had more therapeutic options for taming the symptoms of the menopause. We have an unprecedented understanding of diet and nutrition and the role they play in healthy ageing. Women, although still struggling for equality in many areas, have trampled down many of the old barriers of sexual stereotypes and discrimination. Many women in their 50s are just entering the best years of their professional careers. Attitudes to women and their roles and worth in society are changing, as are attitudes towards the experience of the menopause and those women who are in it.

But this may be a good time to rethink some of your most deep-rooted ideas. This chapter acknowledges and evaluates some of the 'truths' you've learned about the menopause and ageing over the years, and how those ideas can affect your attitude toward your own experience. It also takes a closer look at some of the myths and fears that surround the menopause, even in today's enlightened social climate, and offers some simple techniques for tracking unproductive and unhealthy beliefs to their source and cleaning them out of your mental cupboard. The menopause is a positive experience, and the final sections of this chapter focus on the real benefits you gain as you pass into this phase of your life. It's easy for you to believe the worst about the menopause; now, it's time to see the menopause for what it is – and what it can be.

This Isn't Your Mother's Menopause

If you're 50 years old today – one year younger than the average age of menopause in the UK – you were born sometime around 1955, and (on average), your mother was born between 1925 and 1937. She probably went through the menopause some time in late 1970s or early 1980s. Think about those dates for just a moment and consider how much society has changed during that time. When your mother was born, little was said about the menopause and few women would have felt comfortable talking about 'the change' even within a group of friends. Today, it's not unusual for the menopause to be the subject of happy-hour chatter. So, much of what we say about the menopause has changed – but how about the way we think about the menopause? Has our basic set of ideas and beliefs about the menopause gone through a true evolution in the same way?

What Our Mothers Taught Us

If you ask many women in their 50s today what their mothers told them about the menopause, they're likely to respond, 'She never mentioned it to me.' If society was breaking down the barriers that deemed the menopause an unacceptable topic, why wasn't more information available about the menopause during the 1970s and 1980s?

Much of the lack of new information about the menopause during this time was the result of a shortage of good menopause research prior to the last quarter of the 20th century. In addition, the research that was being conducted wasn't available to the general public; these were pre-internet years, remember, and newspapers and television programmes weren't likely to report new findings in the field of the menopause. For these reasons, many women in the 1970s didn't have access to updated, comprehensive medical information about symptoms, their causes and how they might be alleviated.

Although your mother may have never discussed the menopause with you, that doesn't mean that you – and millions of other women of your generation – didn't 'inherit' certain beliefs about the menopause. Your mother's beliefs about the menopause and the general attitude of the women in her generation towards this important transition could be transferred to you, whether or not those beliefs were spoken. How your mother handled the menopause has almost certainly coloured your attitude towards the menopause – and will, therefore, have some impact upon shaping your own experience.

What Our Mothers Taught Medicine

Since the late 1970s, the medical profession has studied menopausal women more than in any time in history, and what it has learned from those women – a group that includes the mothers of the current generation of those in their 40s and 50s – has changed the way in which science and society view the menopause. Symptoms such as hot flushes, insomnia and irritability were viewed as all-in-the-head responses to the panic of ageing. Today, many scientists trace these symptoms to specific changes in the body's hormone levels. In the 1980s, most women viewed hormone replacement therapy (HRT) as the only option for relieving menopausal symptoms. Today, HRT is just one treatment choice. The world is a different place for today's menopausal women thanks, in part, to data gathered for and by their mothers' generation.

Today, any woman approaching the menopause has a wide variety of health-care resources, treatment options, support groups, information sources and discussion forums to turn to for information, advice and ideas about having a healthy, satisfying transition to the menopause. Menopausal women don't have to 'shut up and get through it' or deny that they're experiencing natural emotional and physical reactions to this important passage.

Today's 50-year-olds have a third of their lives ahead of them. They will live longer than any generation of women that preceded them, and they won't experience this 'Third Age' as their mothers experienced it. To live the years ahead productively and happily, women in this group must come face to face with their body, their health and their attitudes towards making the transition to the menopause.

Common Wisdom: What's It Worth?

Do you remember Health Education or Sex Education classes back in the late 1960s or early 1970s? If so, you undoubtedly recall the plastic model of the female reproductive organs that graced the teacher's desk. At some point in the course, the teacher would send the model around the room, so everyone could get a closer look. The girls would pass the model around, eyeing it casually and handing it to the next student – nothing to see here, folks! The sexual revolution was just unfolding, and young girls were learning to regard their bodies and sexuality in wholly new ways.

In a time of growing sexual freedom, adolescent girls learned to be cool and nonchalant about sexuality – and they certainly weren't caught up in issues their mothers and grandmothers thought of as 'female problems'. They laughed at old euphemisms for menstruation, such as 'that time of the month' or 'getting the curse'. In an age of feminism, these women learned to toss aside the old concepts of feminine weakness and fragility and recognize themselves as strong, capable, free-thinking, sexual creatures.

But now, as they approach the menopause, many women in this post-feminist age are considering their femaleness from another perspective. At some point, every woman begins to contemplate certain facts about this time of transition, and to acknowledge some of the following basic truths:

· Some physical aspects of the ageing process are unique to women;
· The body and mind of a 50-year-old woman are different from those of a 25-year-old woman;
· The menopause marks a physical change in a woman's body, and every woman's reaction to that physical change will be different.

Beyond these simple, basic truths, however, most of us hold a number of ideas and attitudes towards the menopause and ageing – some true and some false. So how do you think about the menopause? Do you dread it? Are you looking forward to the freedom of moving beyond menstruation and into a life free of the possibility of unwanted pregnancy? Or do you equate fertility with femininity, and worry that the menopause will leave you dried up and dreary? Are you hopeful that with the right diet, treatment plan and nutritional supplements you can get back the body you had at 25? Or at least keep the one you have at 45? Do you know the woman you are, and can you accept the woman you are becoming?

Your attitude toward the menopause and the ageing process will determine the answers to many of these questions. And the first step in understanding how you feel about the menopause is to examine the source of those feelings and ideas.

The common wisdom of the menopause – the information and misinformation that fuel society's beliefs – plays an important role in determining what we believe. We may know that a widely held belief is simply untrue, but it's easier to sort fact from fiction when we take a moment to understand the nugget of truth that may have blossomed into a full-blown myth. So take a moment to review some of the beliefs below that make up the common wisdom of the menopause, so that you can understand the truths – and untruths – they hold.

Menopausal Women Lose Interest in Sex

The lack-of-libido mythology about women in the menopause is part of the common wisdom shared by both men and women – and it's simply not true. Masters and Johnson conducted a study that demonstrated no link between oestrogen levels and libido. A number of studies have shown that only a small percentage of postmenopausal women report a lack of interest in sex, and over half of all women studied report no decrease in sexual interest at all after the menopause. In fact, a recent sexual survey, conducted in 1999, showed that over two-thirds of men and women aged 45 and older say they're satisfied with their sex lives, and many say they enjoy sex 'now more than ever'.

So where did this myth come from? The truth is that women suffering from severe oestrogen depletion can experience some discomfort during sex due to drier, thinner, less flexible vaginal walls and occasional itching and burning near the vaginal opening. A woman experiencing hot flushes, disturbed sleep patterns, headaches and other occasional symptoms of the menopause is unlikely to feel as sexually eager as she would otherwise. However, none of these conditions is permanent or untreatable, and many of them aren't inevitable, either. So, if you believe that the menopause equals the end of sex as you know it, you're wrong.

Women in Menopause Gain Weight, Have Hot Flushes and Lose Control of Their Emotions

Lots of people think that the typical woman in the menopause is fat, flushed and out of control. While hot flushes, weight gain and mood swings are all symptoms reported by some women in they menopause, they aren't inevitable side effects of the passage. In fact, many women – as many as 10 to 20 per cent of women studied – exhibit no symptoms of the menopause at all. And while studies show that as many as half of all women in the perimenopause experience some weight gain, other women actually lose weight during the perimenopause; and many of those who gain weight before the menopause lose it afterward. (See Chapters 13 and 14 for information about weight management in the menopause.)

Perhaps as many as 85 per cent of menopausal women report hot flushes, but most women find them to be intermittent and, on average, they diminish completely within five years after the menopause. (See Chapter 16.)

Irritability and depression are also symptoms reported by some – but not all – women during the perimenopause, but no one should expect depression to be a long-term, ongoing fact of life during this transition. In fact, depression is reported at much higher rates among women in their 20s and 30s, and some studies have shown that depression actually decreases in postmenopausal women. And even if you do experience mood swings, they don't have to become part of your identity during the menopause. (See Chapter 18.)

In short, you may or may not have hot flushes, moodiness and weight gain during the menopause – many women don't. But if you do experience these symptoms, they are likely to be temporary and can be treated by a number of therapeutic options.

Hormone Replacement Therapy Is Dangerous

Almost 35 per cent of women in the menopause use some form of hormone replacement therapy (HRT). It's true that HRT can have dangerous consequences for women with a history of breast cancer, blood clots, endometrial cancer and certain other family health concerns.

No reputable doctor would prescribe HRT for a woman whose health history indicates that it may be harmful for her. But most doctors agree that HRT is one of the most effective methods available today for minimizing both the uncomfortable symptoms (such as hot flushes and vaginal dryness) and health-threatening side effects (including elevated cholesterol levels and bone loss) of the menopause. Still, many women continue to view HRT as a treatment option pushed by doctors as a means of making money for both the medical profession and the pharmaceutical industry.

Many of the studies that indicated links between oestrogen and endometrial cancer were conducted on women who were given oestrogen alone, without the balancing hormone progesterone, in the early days of HRT. Today, doctors prescribe both hormones for women who still have a uterus. Women who take both hormones actually have a lower risk of endometrial cancer than women who take no hormones. And other studies show that the benefits of HRT, including reduced heart disease, improved blood cholesterol levels and lowered incidences of osteoporosis, far outweigh the risks.

Many, many studies on the benefits and potential health implications of HRT are underway, and new reports appear regularly. To keep up with some of the latest news about HRT, you can view the British Menopause Society's website at *www.the-bms.org*, or alternatively go to *www.nhsdirect* and look up 'menopause' or 'HRT'.

You may or may not be a good candidate for HRT, and you can certainly use other methods for treating symptoms. If you do decide to use HRT, you may take it for only a short period of time. To know and understand your options, read as much as you can on the topic and talk to your doctor and other health-care professionals. But keep an open mind, listen to the facts and learn all you can about HRT. (See Chapter 11 for more information.) Then make your decision based on fact – not fear.

HRT Is the Only Viable Option for Dealing with the Symptoms of the Menopause

HRT isn't the only option for treating menopause symptoms or delaying the ageing effects of slowing oestrogen production. Depending upon the symptoms you experience, simple lifestyle changes may address your most annoying reminders of the perimenopause. During your mother's experience with the menopause, HRT was just about the only treatment option discussed with women in the transition. So many women in that generation faced an HRT-or-nothing choice. But the truths about the menopause have changed dramatically over the past 30 years.

What exactly are alternative treatments for symptoms of the menopause?
Alternative treatments are any treatment other than the traditional treatment of hormone replacement therapy. Alternative treatments include anything from vitamins and herbs, to nutritional supplements of soya and phyto-oestrogens, to cognitive therapy, acupuncture and biofeedback.

As women have learned more about the causes and life cycles of certain menopausal symptoms, they feel more comfortable tackling some of them with simple lifestyle changes. You can sleep in a cool bedroom and wear layers of clothing to combat hot flushes, for example. Relaxation therapies can help reduce the occurrence of insomnia, as can changes in eating and drinking habits. If you suffer from anxiety and depression, you might benefit from psychological counselling or biofeedback therapy. A number of herbal remedies, prescription and over-the-counter medications and dietary supplements are available to help fight off bone loss, high cholesterol, sleeplessness and other menopause-related health concerns. Women who cannot or prefer not to use oestrogen can choose from a number of sound, viable non-HRT treatment options for combatting the symptoms of the menopause.

Menopausal Women Are Angry, Bitter and Old

You need only to look around you to see through this lie. First, the average age of the menopause in the United Kingdom is 51 – hardly an age that anyone in today's society (anyone over the age of 20) would view as being old. And some women go through the menopause – even natural menopause – in their 40s. There's a big difference between growing older and being 'old'. And who has time to be bothered about chronology, anyway? It's how old you *feel* that counts.

Beyond that, few women in this society have lives that grind to a halt when their reproductive system slows down. Women's lives aren't defined by the number of children sitting around their supper table each evening, and the empty nest more often than not evolves into a house full of other interests and opportunities. Many women are just entering the most productive and lucrative stages of their careers during and after the menopause, and find that their career satisfaction actually increases at this time. The menopause can be a time of unprecedented self-confidence, freedom and financial liberation for women. Anger and bitterness aren't a natural and inevitable side effect of the transition.

The menopause is a time of reflection, though. For many women, the menopause is a time of introspection and personal assessment. Some women have spent the majority of their lives preceding the menopause caring for other people and interests – children, spouses or partners, parents and careers. If these women turn more attention inwards, their behaviour might on the surface make them appear to be withdrawn or even angry. The menopause is a time of change, and for many women that change extends deeper than the rhythm of their ovarian cycles. Blanket assumptions about the feelings and attitudes of menopausal women – or women of any age, for that matter – are never accurate.

Constructing Your Own Common Wisdom

The previous sections discuss only a few of the commonly held misconceptions about the experience of the perimenopause and menopause. While these examples help illustrate how wrong these generalities can be, many other inaccuracies dominate the popular culture about the menopause and what it means to go through it. Common wisdom exists because it's easier to accept a set of broad generalizations than it is to dig out the facts of any issue or idea. But when it comes to the subject of the menopause, generalities that apply in the majority of cases simply don't exist.

Every woman's experience in the menopause will differ. And yours is really the only experience that matters to you. If you keep an open mind and pay attention to your own body and the facts about menopause it teaches you, you'll find your own set of common wisdom truths about this transition and what it means for you. If you monitor and respond to your own body's reactions, and discuss your concerns openly and thoroughly with your doctor, you'll be better able to make the best lifestyle and health-care decisions for you during your passage through the menopause.

Your Chances for a Brand New Start

If women in the past thought of the menopause as the beginning of the end, more and more women today are seizing upon this time of transition as an opportunity to make important changes in their lifestyles and behaviour. As mentioned earlier, many women devote their premenopausal adult years to focusing outwards, on the demands of family, finances and careers. As a woman approaches the menopause, however, her life may offer her many new opportunities for personal freedom and growth. Many postmenopausal women find that their families and home life actually improve at this time, and that they have a greater sense of personal fulfillment.

With less time spent caring for young children or developing first-time relationships with husbands or partners, or gaining a foothold in the workplace, postmenopausal women can devote more time to their personal interests. Women find new energy and interest in returning to pursuits they abandoned in their 20s and 30s, including creative outlets such as painting, writing and photography. Many women at the age of the menopause find themselves able to devote time and energy to travel, finishing an abandoned academic degree or starting a new business.

The menopause is a time when many women make important lifestyle changes. During most of your life, you may not have worried much about issues such as nutrition and exercise or the health-threatening impact of smoking, living with stress or inadequate sleep. But as you approach the age of the menopause, you may find that you're ready to make changes in your habits now, in order to ensure a happier, healthy future. In fact, although the stereotype of age may be that it's a time of reminiscence and living in the past, many women find themselves contemplating the future more than ever as they approach the menopause. Although you may be nearing the end of your reproductive years, your non-reproductive productivity may achieve levels you've never known.

Part of the freedom of the menopause is that it gives women an opportunity to define themselves in terms of who they are, rather than how well they fit the stereotype of what women are 'supposed' to be. Many women spend their youth attempting to fulfill the popular culture's ideal of what a woman should be: thin, beautiful, neat, industrious, helpful, tireless and supportive of family, friends, supervisor, parents and anyone else that she encounters in her day. In other words, she's a mother, a partner and a helper. Women in the menopause have an opportunity to throw down that identity and discover what they want, what they enjoy and how they can best fulfill their needs.

In her book *The Wisdom of Menopause*, Dr Christiane Northrup stresses that most menopausal women do grieve past losses. When you're no longer a young mother, a young wife or a 'fresh young face' at the office, you realize that one identity is passing, even as another begins. But Dr Northrup contends that the biggest message the menopause brings women is not one of loss; rather, the menopause is a wake-up call, 'as each woman struggles to make a new life, one that can accommodate her emerging self'.

Since you were born, you have been in a constant state of growth and change. Through the years, your attitudes and beliefs have helped to determine how well you fared in each stage of your life. Your ability to adapt to change, to take advantage of opportunities that came your way and to capitalize on the realities of your situation have determined the successes or failures you've enjoyed – in both your personal and professional lives. That's why your attitudes and beliefs about the menopause matter.

As part of the largest generation of post-50-year-old women in history, you have the opportunity to help shape the common wisdom about what postmenopausal women are all about. Deciding to be well-informed and active in the maintenance of your future health and happiness is the surest way toward a good experience with the menopause and a healthy, fulfilling postmenopausal life.

Don't imagine that healthy introspection has to lead to an it's-all-about-me attitude. There's a big difference between self-evaluation and self-absorption. Instead, think of your Third Age as an opportunity to become reacquainted with yourself – who you are and what your dreams are, now. This time of self-realization and discovery can benefit both you and your relationships with others.

CHAPTER 5

Working with Your Doctor

In an age where traditional and alternative health-care go hand in hand, few women go through their adult lives with one single health practitioner. The increased mobility of modern life has served to do away with the lifetime family doctor, too. That's why it's important for every woman to participate actively in the management of her own health.

Do You Have the Doctor You Need Now?

The chance that you'll see the same health-care professional at the age of 50 that you saw at 20 grows slimmer with each passing day. You need to be an active partner in your health maintenance throughout your life; if you have been a passive patient up to this point, now's the time to get serious and get involved in ensuring your good health throughout the menopause – and beyond.

During the perimenopause and menopause, your health care needs differ from those when you were younger. You may begin experiencing abnormalities in your menstrual cycle, such as irregular or heavy bleeding. Your symptoms could be caused by hormonal fluctuations of approaching menopause – or by serious diseases, such as pre-cancerous changes in the lining of the uterus or even endometrial cancer. You may need diagnosis and treatment of emotional as well as physical symptoms. And you most certainly will need the medical advice of someone who is up-to-date on medical advancements in menopause symptoms and treatment, knowledgeable about a range of treatment options, and willing and able to discuss those options with you. Even if you've been pretty casual about health care during your 20s, 30s and early 40s, the approach of the menopause signals an end to ho-hum health care. Your health care actions and choices now can determine the quality of the rest of your life.

You may have a great GP right now, or you may need to begin your search for a GP who's right for you. In either case, now is the time to evaluate what you want and need in a health-care provider, and to make sure that you have the man or woman who fulfills that role.

The first step in choosing the right health care provider for your menopause journey is to determine what kind of person you want to work with.

If you have the opportunity to choose your GP – which is rare in this day and age – then consider the following:

· Would you rather see see a male or a female doctor? You're going to need to be comfortable with this person, so you need to decide if gender plays a role in your willingness to discuss symptoms, lifestyle factors and treatment alternatives. If you'll feel reluctant to be totally open and honest with a doctor because of his or her gender, this may not be the time to try to break down those barriers.

- Do you feel comfortable with a medical 'boss' who will dispense advice and guidance without requesting your input regarding treatment options? Or would you prefer someone who is open to the patient-as-partner approach to health care?
- Do you care about the age of your GP? Again, it's important that you feel comfortable with your doctor, you're willing to openly discuss your health and lifestyle issues, and you're confident in the decisions and recommendations that you're offered.

Alternative Practitioners

Mentioned below are just a few types of complementary therapies you might consult during the menopause. For a more complete discussion of alternative treatments for symptoms of the menopause, see Chapter 12. Many women use alternative medicine techniques to combat symptoms of the menopause in conjunction with traditional medicine. If you're interested in exploring both traditional and alternative medical approaches to treating your menopause symptoms, make sure any doctor you use is open to helping you as you pursue this approach.

- Herbalists prescribe herbal supplements and treatments to combat symptoms of the menopause. Herbal remedies are growing in popularity in Western cultures, and many women today turn to herbs such as black cohosh, evening primrose and gingko biloba to offset symptoms such as hot flushes, insomnia and memory loss. Herbal substances are not benign treatment alternatives, however, and herbalists are trained to help determine the best types, amounts and delivery mechanisms for herbal treatment of menopause symptoms.
- Homeopaths offer a type of medical treatment that operates on the principle that like cures like. Homeopaths prescribe small doses of substances that, if not diluted, would actually make symptoms worse; homeopathic prescription amounts are based on the severity of symptoms, rather than the age and weight of the patient.

'Natural' doesn't mean 'safe'. Though you can purchase many over-the-counter herbal supplements for relief of menopausal symptoms, you need to be very careful in their use. Many plants and herbs deliver significant doses of oestrogen or interact with other supplements and prescription drugs. Check with your doctor or health-care provider before embarking on any type of treatment.

- Acupuncturists use a 2,000-year-old treatment technique that involves rotating fine, sterilized needles into the patient's skin to bring about a therapeutic response. Many women in the menopause turn to acupuncture for relief of such symptoms as headaches, anxiety, insomnia and fatigue.

Getting the Best from Your GP

Finding a good doctor is only half of the sound menopause management equation. In order to make the best decisions and follow the best lifestyle decisions and treatment approaches, you need to be an active, informed, involved partner in the management of your health care. You're reading this book, which suggests that you understand the importance of becoming well informed about menopause issues, symptoms and treatment options. Use the information you read here (and in the recommended resources listed in Appendix B) to decide what kinds of questions and options you want to explore with your GP. The following sections discuss some simple ways you can prepare to be a good patient who brings out the best in her good doctor.

If you're seeing a doctor or alternative practitioner about issues related to the menopause, you aren't a child any more. As obvious as that seems, it's important that you drop a lot of the passive techniques you may have developed when dealing with doctors (and other authority figures) in your youth. If you've followed the advice given up to this point in the chapter, you've spent a lot of time and energy tracking down the right doctor or alternative practitioner to help you deal most effectively with the symptoms and biological and physiological effects of the menopause. So do your GP a favour, and approach any consultation as an exchange of information – not a tell-me-what-to-do-and-I'll-leave event.

During your first appointment, the doctor will ask you a number of questions regarding your individual and family health histories. As a rule, you'll need to report on any personal and family history of blood clots, heart disease, breast cancer and osteoporosis, among other conditions. Your doctor will also ask you about your current medications – both over-the-counter and prescription drugs – as well as your use of alcohol, recreational drugs and tobacco. You're not running for school head girl here, so don't attempt to whitewash the facts by presenting yourself as you think you should be. If you drink or smoke, say so. And don't forget that over-the-counter medications, such as pain relievers, vitamins, minerals and nutritional supplements, count; report any substances you regularly consume, so your doctor or practitioner can be aware of them when he or she prescribes treatment.

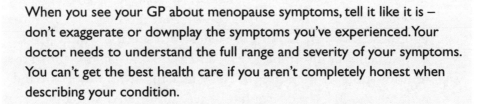

When you see your GP about menopause symptoms, tell it like it is – don't exaggerate or downplay the symptoms you've experienced. Your doctor needs to understand the full range and severity of your symptoms. You can't get the best health care if you aren't completely honest when describing your condition.

During your first visit, remember to mention all symptoms you've been experiencing – both emotional and physical. If your periods have become irregular in any way, report the irregularities. (Take your menstrual calendar to the visit.) Mood swings and depression are important indicators of your current health, as is any change in your interest in sex. If you're suffering from periodic involuntary urine release, report that and explain the conditions. Take a written list of symptoms, questions and concerns with you to your visit, and write down the answers you receive from your GP.

If you've been keeping a menstruation journal or menstrual calendar (see Chapter 3), take it to your initial visit with your doctor. He or she can gain valuable information about your current condition by reviewing even a two- or three-month history of your symptoms. Add to your calendar any symptoms that seem to run in cycles, such as headaches, water retention or unusual pelvic pain.

Before you leave the surgery, make sure you understand all the information you've received. If you need further explanation, ask for it. You won't get points for pretending to understand information that confuses you. If your doctor is using terminology you don't understand, ask for a translation. Many doctors' surgeries also have pre-printed brochures regarding various aspects of the menopause, so feel free to ask.

Finally, discuss all treatment options that interest you. If you're interested in pursuing a combination approach to managing symptoms of the menopause, you want to be certain that this doctor is open to that approach. If you are looking for relief from specific symptoms, such as incontinence or insomnia, say so, and ask if any recommended treatment options specifically address those symptoms. If you think you may want certain tests that the doctor hasn't actually offered, speak up.

Take an Active Role

In order for any therapy to be effective, you must be committed to following it – as directed – for as long as is necessary to gauge its results and effectiveness. Remember, you aren't a passive observer in your journey through the menopause. Being an active partner in your treatment plan involves carefully monitoring your response to therapeutic drugs and treatments, and keeping your GP or alternative health practitioner informed of your progress. If you have a negative reaction to drugs or other treatment options, speak up. You could be experiencing normal adjustment reactions, or you could be embarking on a plan that simply doesn't match your body chemistry, lifestyle or biological and physiological make-up. You won't know what's wrong unless you report the reaction to your doctor.

If you are using a combination of treatment options, make sure that you coordinate all of them with your GP. Maybe you've heard about the benefits of using biofeedback-assisted behavioural training to control urine discharge, and you'd like to explore that option. Before you book a biofeedback session, talk to your GP about the process, to make sure this won't conflict with any other treatments you're pursuing.

Finally, don't remain passively disappointed with your treatment. If you feel unhappy with the health care you're receiving, just say so. Your doctor can't correct a problem that he or she doesn't know about. If you're unhappy with the progress of your symptom-relief treatment, discuss your concerns with your GP. If you feel that your doctor is unresponsive to your questions and concerns, give him or her an opportunity to discuss your feelings. Although you want to build and maintain a respectful relationship with your doctor, choose honesty over diplomacy in this discussion. Be very specific and open as you state your concerns, and listen carefully to the response. If you can't resolve your differences, it's time to start looking for a new GP.

Listen, Speak Up, Be Honest

Throughout this chapter, you're reminded that you carry a big part of the responsibility for making sure that you get the best possible health care. When you've chosen a health-care provider who meets your needs and fits your own list of qualifications, you can't simply sit back and enjoy the ride. To make sure that you help your GP continue to give you the best advice and treatment options during your transition through the perimenopause, remember the following important guidelines:

· Listen to the information your doctor gives you. When you ask a question, take notes of the response if necessary; don't assume that you already know what your GP is going to say. Just listen carefully, and ask further questions if necessary.

- Ask questions, voice concerns, report problems and discuss options; your GP depends upon your active involvement in your health care.
- Be honest. You must be honest in your communications with your doctor. Many people think that they'll annoy their doctor or alternative practitioner by asking too many questions or by discussing issues that they don't fully understand or agree with. Most doctors find it much more challenging to deal with patients who act as though they're OK with a plan or fully understand a treatment option, when that isn't really the case. You can't have good health care if you don't communicate honestly with your health-care provider.

CHAPTER 6

General Health Risks and Management after the Age of 40

I f the first 40 years of your life were spent in blissful ignorance of the toll that each passing year might take on your physical health, now is the time to get serious about your personal maintenance plan. If you are aware of the common health risks that women face after 40, you will know what changes you need to make in your diet and lifestyle.

The Health Risks We Face after 40

First, let's all agree that age isn't a number, and turning 40 doesn't signal an onslaught of health-riddling diseases and disabilities. Many women are healthier than they've ever been as they approach midlife. But a well-thought-out approach to health management and maintenance is wise at any age, and it becomes more important as each year passes. Don't think of your health-care efforts as part of entering old age; think of them as a simple, basic plan to preserve and extend your youth.

Everyone – man and woman – has to invest a bit more time and attention in his or her 'machine' as it ages. Our bodies work hard, and after years of service, even routine maintenance becomes more demanding – and essential. If we reach a stage where our jobs and personal lives have become less physically demanding but, perhaps, more mentally draining, it's easy to overlook the shifting load our bodies must bear. We lose track of the trade we've made in how we spend our time and mental energy, with less time spent outdoors and in fewer physical activities, and more time spent sitting behind desks or in the car, struggling to meet deadlines, resolving problems or sorting out schedules.

Many people enter their 40s sandwiched between caring for their children and parents at the same time. Add to that the accumulation of many years of not-so-healthy habits – basing our nutrition pyramid on sugar, fat and deep-fried anything; smoking; yo-yo-ing from one weight-loss plan to the next; skimping on sleep then counting on caffeine to power us through the day – and it's easy to see why our bodies might need a little TLC as they hit midlife.

For women, though, the physical effects of an ageing reproductive system can present some special health risks. Oestrogen provides women with a natural protection against certain diseases, such as osteoporosis, heart disease and decrease in vaginal secretions. In the perimenopause, because a woman's body produces less oestrogen, she becomes more vulnerable to these and other health risks. Many physical symptoms that might be attributed to the first pangs of ageing might actually be the first warning signals of serious health problems in the making. So a good health-care routine at 40 can lay the groundwork for a healthy passage through 50, 60, 70, 80 and beyond.

The following sections of this chapter look at some of the most common age-related health factors that deserve your attention as you approach the menopause. When you understand the types of health risks and issues you may face, you can begin sketching the outline of your own midlife health management strategy. The 'Your Contribution to Your Health' section of this chapter offers you useful detection and prevention methods that can help you manage these risks as you move towards and through the menopause.

Heart Disease and the Menopause

Heart disease is a term we've all heard, but may not fully understand. The umbrella term covers a wide range of diseases, illnesses and events that affect the heart and circulatory system – known as cardiovascular diseases. High blood pressure and coronary artery disease that can lead to stroke, heart attacks and early death are some of the most common forms of heart disease for both men and women.

We've all grown accustomed to thinking of the typical victim of heart disease as a middle-aged, overweight, out-of-shape man, but that's yet another stereotype that just doesn't reflect the real picture. Heart disease is a major killer of women over 50 in Britain. It's true that prior to the menopause, women suffer fewer effects of heart disease and stroke than men. But as women age, their risk of heart disease increases dramatically.

Some studies indicate that a woman's natural oestrogen loss due to ageing may contribute to heart disease. Oestrogen can help control the body's blood cholesterol levels, and it keeps a woman's total cholesterol low before the menopause, with low levels of LDL (low-density lipoproteins or 'bad' cholesterol) and high levels of the 'good' cholesterol, HDL (high-density lipoproteins). These fractions are reversed after the menopause, and are thought to be serious contributors to one's risk of a heart attack. Women over 55 have higher blood cholesterol levels than men, and women are particularly vulnerable to low levels of HDL.

Over 30,000 deaths a year are caused by obesity in England alone. The condition costs the NHS an estimated £500 million a year. Adult obesity rates have almost quadrupled in the last 25 years. Now 22 per cent of adult Britons are obese, and a staggering three-quarters of us are overweight.

Oestrogen loss isn't the only contributing factor to heart disease and stroke for women as they move through the perimenopause, however. If, as you approach the menopause, you begin putting on weight, particularly around your abdomen (starting to look like an 'apple' instead of a 'pear'), you could be significantly increasing your risk of heart disease. Other midlife diseases, such as diabetes and high blood pressure, are strongly linked to the onset of heart disease in midlife as well.

Too often, heart attacks are misdiagnosed in women with the symptoms attributed to heartburn, indigestion or gallbladder disease. As women move towards the menopause, their risk factors for heart disease increase dramatically, and so their vigilance and heart-healthy habits have to increase to offset the risk. Although family health history plays a role in your own likelihood of developing heart disease, you have many options for combatting this deadly enemy, including diet, exercise, lifestyle changes, cholesterol-controlling medications, HRT and more.

Cancer Risks

Over a third of all women in the UK will develop cancer during their lifetimes, and more than one in four will die from it, so as you approach the menopause, it's important that you understand which cancers have age-related risk factors for women.

Cancer isn't one disease. It is a family of diseases, all of which occur when cell growth goes out of control in some part of the body. Cancer has been widely studied, but its causes are complex and still not fully understood. Contributing factors include environmental pollutants, heredity, occupation, nutrition and lifestyle. At times, there is no medical explanation for why a certain type of cancer develops in a previously healthy person. Different cancers produce very different illnesses, each with its own symptoms, causes and risk factors. The following sections discuss some of the most common cancers that women face as they move into middle age. The object of this information isn't to alarm you or to convince you that you're doomed to suffer from this disease. But knowledge is power; this brief overview gives you information about the risks your health-management plan should monitor.

Lung Cancer

Mortality from breast cancer in the UK has fallen steadily since 1990, probably because of earlier detection and improved treatment. In 2002, lung cancer was the leading cause of cancer death in women in the UK. It caused 18 per cent of deaths; breast cancer caused 17 per cent.

Although neither menopause nor age is a contributing factor in this disease, most women are diagnosed with lung cancer at 50 – just at the time they hit the menopause, and often after 35 or more years of tobacco smoke exposure. Women are twice as likely as men to contract cancer from tobacco smoke, including secondhand smoke – the vast majority of non-smokers who contract lung cancer are women.

If you're approaching menopause, the time is right for you to stop smoking – now. You're approaching a new phase of your life, so why not start it smoke-free? Smoking increases your chances of contracting cervical cancer, emphysema and other life-threatening chronic lung conditions. Any illness you contract will be complicated by the effects of smoking. Smoking is a certain way to derail an active, healthy passage into middle life.

According to Cancer Research UK, giving up smoking results in the following changes:

· after just 20 minutes, your blood pressure and pulse return to normal
· after 8 hours, blood oxygen levels return to normal
· after 24 hours, there is no more carbon monoxide in your body

And, over time, your risk of all the serious diseases caused by smoking is dramatically cut:

· 3 years after stopping, your risk of heart attack is the same as for a non-smoker
· 10 years after stopping, the lung cancer risk is halved
· 15 years after stopping, your health is effectively the same as that of a non-smoker

Nicotine replacement products help many people stop smoking – studies show they can double your chances of success. There are several kinds available, including patches, inhalers, nasal spray, lozenges and gum. You can buy them over the counter, or your GP may prescribe them.

Zyban is a prescription-only non-nicotine treatment in tablet form. It works in the brain to help break the addiction to nicotine. Zyban reduces cravings for cigarettes and reduces withdrawal symptoms. Studies have shown that it doubles your chances of success.

Your GP can tell you about quitting clinics and advice centres in your area. It's usually far easier to give up if you get specialist support.

The national Quitline or NHS smoking helpline offers friendly and expert counselling. If you need encouragement to take the first step, or if you're finding it hard to stay stopped, give them a call.
Quitline: 0800 002200
NHS Smoking helplines:
England & Wales: 0800 1690169
Scotland & Northern Ireland: 0800 848484

Breast Cancer

Breast cancer may not cause as many deaths as lung cancer, but it is the most common cancer in women, accounting for 30 per cent of all new cases. There were more than 40,000 new cases in 2000. Large bowel and lung cancer are the second and third most common cancers in women. These cancers in women account for half of all newly diagnosed cases.

If your mother, sister or daughter has had breast cancer, your risks of contracting it go up two to three times (depending on how many of these first-degree relatives are involved). And if you've had breast cancer before, you have a higher risk of developing it again. If you've never had a child, or had your first child after the age of 30, your risk goes up as well. At the age of 40, a British woman's risk of breast cancer is 1 in 200; at 50 it is 1 in 50; at 60 it is 1 in 23; and over a lifetime it is 1 in 9.

But what about risk factors that you can change? Cancer Research UK lists the following risk factors for breast cancer that are specifically linked to lifestyle choices:

Hormone replacement therapy (HRT): Most large studies and most world experts agree that long-term use of hormones after menopause does not significantly increase your risk of breast cancer, though a few studies suggest that long-term use (ten or more years) of HRT may result in a slight increase in the risk of breast cancer. These conflicting studies have not gone unnoticed, and the connection between breast cancer and HRT is still the subject of ongoing research. Some medical professionals suspect that women on HRT are more likely to do self-breast tests, see their doctors regularly and have mammograms. These women are more likely to have their cancers diagnosed at a very early stage, usually before they can even be palpated by the physician or on a self-breast test, so these tiny cancers can be cured with conservative surgery such as lumpectomy. These women also live longer than their counterparts who take no hormones, presumably due to their regular medical check-ups and the protective effect of oestrogen on the heart.

Alcohol: Women who regularly drink alcohol have a slightly increased risk of contracting breast cancer.

Diet: The connection between obesity and breast cancer risk is still being studied, but research indicates that after the menopause, your risk of contracting breast cancer is greater if you are overweight. How much of this risk is linked to your body fat versus specific dietary fat content is still under debate. Another issue may be that more breast tissue (obese women tend to have bigger breasts) makes it harder to find an early, small cancerous lump, both on test and on mammogram.

Exercise: Although research has begun only recently, early findings reported seem to indicate that even moderate physical activity can lower breast cancer risk. And maintaining good overall physical condition certainly improves your chances of having fewer complications related to medical and surgical treatment for any disease – including breast cancer.

Survival rates for breast cancer are highest when the cancer is detected early. The five-year survival rate (your chance of being alive five years after the diagnosis of cancer is made) is 77 per cent for women whose cancer is caught at an early stage. Early detection helps keep the surgery or other treatment that follows diagnosis as non-invasive and conservative as is possible. Techniques for incorporating breast cancer detection into your general health maintenance plan appear later in this chapter.

Ovarian and Uterine Cancers

In the UK, cancer of the ovary is the most common cancer of the female reproductive organs. Over 6,000 new cases of ovarian cancer were diagnosed in the UK in 2000, and more than 5,000 uterine cancers.

Cancer of the uterus, also known as 'womb cancer', is a fairly common type of cancer. It is the fifth most common cancer in women in the UK. Each year, there are over 5,200 new cases. Uterine cancer is usually relatively easy to treat.

The uterus (womb) is a hollow pear-shaped organ located between the bladder and rectum in a woman's pelvis. When a woman becomes pregnant, the foetus develops in the uterus. Most cancers of the uterus develop from cells lining its inner surface. This lining is called the endometrium. Endometrial cancer can spread to other parts of the body.

A number of factors can contribute to the development of uterine cancer:

Age

The risk of endometrial cancer increases with age. Most cancers occur in women after the menopause.

Oestrogen replacement therapy

Having had hormone replacement therapy (HRT) that did not contain progesterone may increase the risk of endometrial cancer.

Obesity

Being overweight can increase the risk of endometrial cancer. This may be because surplus fat will produce more oestrogen.

Tamoxifen therapy

There is an increased risk of endometrial cancer for women who are being treated with tamoxifen for breast cancer. However, the risk is very small. The proven benefits of taking tamoxifen far outweigh the risk of developing endometrial cancer.

Family history

Some people inherit a higher than average risk of endometrial cancer. Members of their family may have been diagnosed with cancer of the bowel, stomach, ovary or endometrium.

Childbearing and menopause

Women who have never been pregnant are more likely to develop endometrial cancer than women with children. Similarly, women who go through their menopause after the age of 52 may have an increased risk.

Personal history of breast or bowel (colorectal) cancer

Women who have had any of these cancers have a greater risk of developing endometrial cancer than other women do.

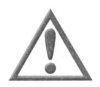

If you have had breast or ovarian cancer, you may have an increased risk for developing endometrial cancer. Some of the same risk factors contribute to all of these forms of cancer, so with the diagnosis of one, your doctor will also monitor you closely for these other cancer types.

If endometrial cancer is diagnosed early, it has a five-year survival rate of 73 per cent. Pre-cancerous changes, such as endometrial hyperplasia, often become known through unusual spotting, bleeding or discharge. Often these symptoms are apparent for years before actual cancer develops. Sometimes women have had irregular periods for their entire lives, and forget to report this to their doctor. Besides, when you're entering the menopause, irregular bleeding, spotting and discharges aren't supposed to be unusual occurrences at all, so how do you know when to worry that your irregularity is signalling endometrial cancer?

Unfortunately, cervical smears – which are great at detecting cervical cancer – don't reveal endometrial cancer. And many women assume that a normal cervical smear result is an assurance of perfect gynaecological health. If you suffer from unusual bleeding that lasts more than two weeks, consult your doctor right away – no matter what your medical history. An endometrial biopsy can determine whether or not your symptoms point to endometrial cancer or some other cause.

Many symptoms of benign conditions, such as fibroids and polyps (uterine growths common in the menopause), are similar to those of endometrial cancer. This 'symptom mimic' makes it even more important that you report any change from what you consider normal for you to your doctor.

Ovarian cancer occurs most often in women who are approaching the age of menopause. This cancer is a silent killer with symptoms that can be mild, vague and similar to those of many other conditions and diseases. If detected early, while still in the ovary, this cancer is curable about

90 per cent of the time. But if the cancer spreads to the pelvis or beyond, the five-year survival rate drops dramatically. Taking all stages into consideration, this cancer's overall five-year survival rate is somewhere around 36 per cent.

Sadly, early ovarian cancer has few symptoms, so it makes sense to know your risk factors and your family history. Risk factors for ovarian cancer include:

· A family history of ovarian, breast, colon, rectal, endometrial or pancreatic cancer increases a woman's risks considerably. The severity of increased risk is higher if there has been one of these cancers in a first-degree relative, such as a mother, sister or daughter.
· A woman's risk of developing ovarian cancer also rises with the total number of times she has ovulated; again, exposure to oestrogen has an impact on the woman's overall risks. In other words, not having had any children or not taking birth-control pills at any point in your life means your ovaries have been working overtime, compared to women in the average population.

Symptoms of ovarian cancer are vague, especially in the early stage, but can include pain, pressure or swelling in your abdomen; wind, nausea and indigestion; unexplained changes in your bowel movements; changes in your weight; fatigue; or pain during intercourse. If you exhibit any of these symptoms, talk to your doctor. He or she can refer you for an ultrasound examination of the pelvis to determine whether your ovaries have any abnormalities.

Fibroids, Polyps and Other Sources of Heavy or Irregular Bleeding

Irregular bleeding isn't uncommon during the perimenopause. Because you ovulate less frequently during this time, your body's oestrogen levels often are unchecked by progesterone. As a result, your uterine lining can develop abnormal cell changes that lead to unusually heavy bleeding or spotting.

As you've learned, irregular bleeding can have a number of causes, but two relatively common benign causes are fibroids and polyps. Fibroids are benign growths of muscle tissue that develop within the wall of the uterus, on the uterine lining or on the outside of the uterus. Two out of five women in their 40s can expect to develop these growths.

Fibroids within the uterine lining can cause abnormal bleeding because of the way they distort the lining and prevent it from shedding normally. Fibroids can sometimes become quite large. Their sheer size alone can cause problems, such as pelvic discomfort, bloating or pain during intercourse. If you have unusually heavy or midcycle bleeding, your doctor probably will check for the presence of fibroids.

Fibroids usually shrink after menopause. As a result, your doctor may or may not choose to treat them with surgery or drugs, depending upon the severity of your symptoms. Conservative treatment options are now also available, usually done as out-patient surgery – a hysteroscopy. In this sophisticated dilation and curettage (D and C) procedure, a tiny camera lens and instrument port are inserted into the cervix to locate the polyps and remove all of them at that time. Although pain is usually minimal, you may request mild sedation during the procedure and analgesics afterwards.

Polyps are smaller benign growths on the lining of the uterus. Science and medicine have yet to explain why polyps develop in some women and not in others. Polyps bleed, just like fibroids, but because they typically are small, they're unlikely to cause the amount of blood loss associated with fibroids. When a doctor diagnoses polyps (usually through an ultrasound test or a biopsy sample), he or she can remove them through a simple out-patient procedure in which the doctor snips the polyps from the uterine lining. This procedure usually involves a hysteroscopy, similar to that used to remove fibroids.

A common cause of abnormal bleeding is a precancerous condition of the lining of the uterus – endometrial hyperplasia. This excessive growth of the uterine lining can result from relatively low levels of progesterone. If diagnosed when still in its early stages, it can be treated medically. Untreated endometrial hyperplasia can develop into endometrial cancer.

The least common cause of irregular bleeding is cancer. But, because endometrial cancer can masquerade as common irregular or heavy menstrual bleeding, it's important to talk to your doctor when your periods become too heavy or too frequent, or vary noticeably from your own personal norm.

Osteoporosis and Age

Osteoporosis – the loss of bone mass that results in porous, fragile bones – is quite common in Britain. Each year there are around 70,000 hip, 120,000 spine and 50,000 wrist fractures due to osteoporosis. Most of these fractures are preventable if a doctor diagnoses the early stages of osteoporosis, called osteopenia, at a time when preventable measures are possible.

Oestrogen helps prevent the loss of bone density, and that's what makes osteoporosis such a growing threat for menopausal women. Hip fractures, crumbling vertebrae (the small bones that make up your spine) and the familiar stooped posture of many elderly women are just some of the all-too-common effects of this disease.

Bone loss begins early; by 35, your body begins to lose more bone material than it generates. Although at that age this decline is very gradual, the loss of bone material speeds up dramatically as oestrogen levels drop off during the perimenopause. In the five to seven years that follow the menopause, the average woman can lose up to 20 per cent of her bone mass, which usually signals the onset of osteoporosis.

The first outright symptom of osteoporosis may be a fractured hip or crumbled vertebrae that happens as the result of no more than a mild bump. Unfortunately, by the time such a break occurs, the disease has already done a lot of damage to your body's framework. Doctors have to depend on family medical history and sound prevention methods to stop osteoporosis before it strikes. Beyond age and the low oestrogen levels that may be present in the perimenopause, risk factors for osteoporosis include a family history of the disease; a small, thin frame; a diet low in calcium; or a history of eating disorders such as anorexia or bulimia (in which oestrogen levels usually drop and menstrual periods often cease).

Smoking, excessive use of alcohol and lack of exercise can contribute to osteoporosis as well.

Some medications, such as corticosteroids, thyroid hormone replacement medications and anticonvulsants, can contribute to bone loss. If your doctor prescribes these medications, be sure you have discussed your family health history and personal risks for osteoporosis.

By the time you've reached the perimenopause, you've passed the age when you could continue to develop a stronger, healthier skeleton. Your goals now should be to slow calcium loss and maintain your bones' current strength. A healthy diet that's rich in calcium, plenty of weight-bearing exercise, and regular bone testing are just some of the ways you can maintain good bone health after menopause. (See Chapter 8 for more information on diagnosis, treatment and prevention options.)

Urinary Tract Disorders and Yeast Infections

During perimenopause, about 40 per cent of women experience some form of urogenital changes – changes to the vagina, genitals and urinary tract. The most common of these changes result from reduction of moisture and elasticity in the vagina that results from depleted oestrogen levels. The vaginal tissue is more easily irritated and broken, and therefore more prone to infections such as vaginitis, yeast infections and urinary tract infections (UTIs). The severity of these disorders ranges from mildly irritating to very painful.

Many women have experienced some type of vaginitis (a swollen, red, irritated vaginal area) at some point in life. These infections include bacterial vaginosis, yeast infections and trichomoniasis. During the perimenopause, fluctuating hormone levels can contribute to the frequency and severity of these infections. Bacteria in the vagina, obesity, diabetes and antibiotics are other contributors. The symptoms of these vaginal infections include burning and itching in the vaginal area, and a discharge.

If you've had yeast infections before and are relatively certain that you're suffering from this type of infection, you can use any of the available over-the-counter creams and other treatments. But if you experience new or unusual symptoms, or the symptoms continue or recur (especially after using an over-the-counter medication), see your doctor for a full diagnosis and treatment. And although you can't prevent all vaginal infections, here are some ways to try to avoid them:

· Don't wear tight clothes (such as jeans) that block air circulation to your lower body, and don't wear pants to bed at night.
· Wear underwear and tights with cotton crotches (avoid tights if you can).
· Be clean, clean, clean; wash your genital area thoroughly, front to back, every day, but...
· Stay away from heavily perfumed and deodorizing soaps, douches, sprays, tampons and pads, and use white unscented toilet paper. All those perfumes and deodorant chemicals can dry out your skin and contribute to acid-level imbalances in your vagina that can then lead to infections.

Fewer layers of clothing are better than too many (although layering the clothes on your upper body is a good idea when you suffer from hot flushes); looser is better than too tight; and natural fabrics such as cotton are better than Lycra and other synthetic fibres. After exercising, swimming or otherwise working up a sweat, change out of sweaty clothes and get into something clean and dry.

If vaginal dryness is a problem for you, your doctor might recommend more frequent sex as a treatment! Sexual arousal – including from masturbation – is a great way to help keep your vaginal tissues moist and flexible.

Urinary tract infections (UTIs) are common in women of all ages, but can be particularly persistent following menopause. In addition to the susceptibility of thin, dry vaginal tissue to infection, the lactobacilli organisms that help fight off bacterial infections in the vagina decline after the menopause. And as the bladder muscles weaken with age, the bladder doesn't empty completely, which can contribute to the build-up of bacteria. UTIs, including cystitis and urethritis, are caused by bacteria (usually from skin around the anus) travelling through the urethra and reaching the bladder or even the kidneys. These bacteria trigger infections that result in symptoms such as pain or burning during urination; sudden, strong and frequent urges to urinate; fever and chills; and even pain in your back, side or abdomen.

The symptoms of more complicated UTIs may vary. If untreated, the bacteria from the bladder can rise to the kidneys. If you have painful urination, accompanied by pain in your back and fever, you may have a kidney infection. Kidney infections can result in chronic and even life-threatening consequences if untreated, so call your doctor immediately if you have these symptoms. If you have painful and quite frequent urination, you may have a bladder infection (commonly known as cystitis). Again, these infections can grow much worse if untreated, so you need to contact your doctor if you experience them. Sometimes more than one course of antibiotics or a different type of antibiotic is necessary to completely eradicate the bacteria.

If recurrent UTIs or symptoms that resemble UTIs become a problem for you, your doctor might recommend oestrogen cream or HRT to help rejuvenate your vaginal tissue. The oestrogen helps increase the blood circulation to this area and restores natural secretions, thus making the entire vagina less susceptible to trauma. But you might be able to avoid some of these infections or discomforts through some simple, healthy regular habits:

· Wipe from front to back, so you don't push bacteria from your anus over your vaginal tissue.
· Drink lots of fluids (water is best) and urinate frequently to keep your urethra (the opening to the bladder) flushed out.

- Keep your vaginal area clean and chemical-free; wash your genital area daily, and avoid any feminine hygiene products that contain additional chemicals, such as deodorant tampons, sanitary pads and panty liners.
- Practice clean, safe sex, and always urinate after sex to flush bacteria from your urethra. It's a good idea for both partners to wash hands and genitals before having sex.
- Use a water-based lubricant such as KY Jelly (rather than an oil-based product such as Vaseline) to reduce friction during intercourse.

Your Contribution to Your Health

Medicine can't do it all. You have to take responsibility for the most important part of your health maintenance – healthy living. Some components of a sensible post-40 health life plan go without saying; but let's list them, anyway:

- Eat a varied diet that's high in vegetables, fruit and complex carbohydrates, and plenty of calcium, vitamins and minerals (see Chapter 13).
- Drink lots of water – at least one litre – every day.
- Exercise regularly – 30 minutes a day, four or more days a week is a minimum recommendation, but every day is better, and any exercise is better than none. Include both weight-bearing and aerobic exercise in your plan (see Chapter 14).
- Stop smoking. Stop smoking. Stop smoking.
- Relax. Stress and fatigue contribute to a wide variety of illnesses and diseases, in ways that we probably don't even fully comprehend. A calm, rested body and mind are your best defence against illness and disease.
- If you're sexually active, get your partner to use a condom and continue using contraception. Remember, until you've been diagnosed as having gone through the menopause (by either an FSH test or after having passed an entire year without a menstrual period), you are still fertile and can still get pregnant.

· Attend any health appointments scheduled for you, such as smear tests or mammograms.

Breast self-exams are your first line of defence against breast cancer. Ask your practice nurse or GP to demonstrate how to check your breasts for lumps or growths; your surgery may provide a leaflet with a visual guide explaining what to do. Self-tests must be accompanied by three-yearly mammograms after the age of 40, especially when you have a cancer-positive family history.

According to Cancer Research UK, the best thing is to be breast-aware. Breasts change in size and shape during the monthly menstrual cycle and at different times in a woman's life. It's important to get to know what your breasts feel like at different times of the month. That way you are more likely to spot an unusual change. Things to look out for are:

* changes in the outline or shape of the breast
* any puckering or dimpling of the skin
* discomfort or pain in one breast, especially if it's new and persists
* lumps or bumpy areas in the breast or armpit that are different from the same area in the other breast or armpit
* nipple discharge that is not milky, bleeding or sore areas that do not heal, and changes in the nipple position or rashes.

There are many reasons for changes in the breast and most of them are harmless, but it's important that they are checked out by a doctor.

CHAPTER 7

The Menopause and Heart Disease

Although it's the number-one killer of women today, few women would name heart disease as a major health concern. The problems that contribute to heart disease can grow silently over a number of years. Even the first signs of serious heart illness, such as a heart attack or stroke, can be attributed to other causes and therefore go unrecognized.

What Is Heart Disease?

The term heart disease refers to any disorder or condition of the heart and blood vessels; these diseases fall under the catch-all category of cardiovascular disease. Coronary artery disease is a common form of heart disease that occurs when arteries become lined with heavy deposits of plaque – a substance made up of fat, calcium and other minerals. The build-up of plaque narrows the diameter of the vessels, thus limiting the amount of blood that can flow through the arteries, contributing to a condition known as atherosclerosis. Blood carries oxygen to all of the body's muscles, including the heart. As plaque narrows or blocks the coronary arteries, the heart is starved of oxygen, which can lead to a heart attack – and damage the heart muscle itself.

Atherosclerosis can also contribute to the plaque build-up in the carotid arteries that carry oxygen-rich blood to the brain. The plaque build-up can lead to the formation of blood clots, which can break loose from the inside of the vessel walls and be carried to your brain, causing a stroke.

Other heart diseases include congestive heart failure, diseases of the heart valves, irregular heartbeats (arrhythmias) and congenital heart diseases. But for women entering the menopause, the threat of heart disease comes mainly from coronary artery disease, the atherosclerosis that contributes to it, and the heart attacks and stroke that all of these conditions can lead to.

The Symptoms of Heart Disease

Unfortunately, coronary artery disease can reach an advanced state without ever issuing a warning sign or symptom. The first major symptom you're likely to experience is a chest pain called angina – a squeezing, heaviness or tightness in your chest that happens when your heart is starved of oxygen. You might feel this pain when you're exercising, climbing stairs or rushing to a meeting, or when you're feeling stressed out or highly emotional. At first, the feeling may be just a momentary pressure that passes quickly if you stop and rest for a moment. However, as the arteries become narrower, you're likely to feel the pain again, and it may radiate down your left arm and shoulder, up through your neck and jaw or down your back. As the atherosclerosis progresses, the pain of angina can become worse. Angina is your warning that you have heart disease and are at risk of suffering a heart attack.

On the other hand, you may have no warning at all. Many people are unaware that they suffer from any kind of heart disease until they have a heart attack, but women are more likely than men to experience the warning pangs of angina before a full heart attack occurs. Because the symptoms of angina are very much like those of a heart attack, it's critical that you report those symptoms to your doctor immediately so that a diagnosis can be made.

When a Heart Attack Hits

If one or more of your coronary arteries becomes completely blocked, you can have a heart attack. A heart attack can be mild, moderate or severe, depending upon the amount of damage to the heart muscle. If only a small area of the heart is deprived of blood, the healthy heart tissue surrounding it continues to work, allowing the damaged part of the heart to heal as new vessels grow in from the healthy areas. But if damage occurs in several of these small areas, they can combine to damage the heart beyond repair.

The symptoms of heart attack vary; in some cases, the attack is so minor that no noticeable symptoms occur. In fact, many heart attacks in women are misdiagnosed as indigestion. But in many other cases, the symptoms of heart attack are evident; we just need to recognize them. Those symptoms include:

· A crushing or dull pain in the chest
· Pain in the left shoulder, arm, neck or back
· Sweating, nausea, shortness of breath

- Fatigue or dizziness
- Burning pain in the midchest area similar to heartburn or indigestion

Heart attacks affect different women in different ways. If you have more than one heart attack, your second one may feel different from the first. That's why it's important that you watch for all signs of heart attack – don't be too quick to dismiss any of them as normal aches and pains.

Only rarely do heart attacks cause the heart to stop functioning completely. More often you have a chance to make a big difference in the amount of damage your heart receives and your chances for a recovery. But you must act quickly; most heart attack damage occurs within the first two hours after you feel the pain. If you have any reason to suspect you may be having an attack – a personal history of angina or a family history of heart disease – be prepared to get help. Sit or lie down for a minute or two. If you continue to feel the symptoms, dial 999 and tell the operator you might be having a heart attack. Then follow that operator's instructions until the ambulance arrives. For example, the operator is likely to ask you to take an aspirin as you wait for the paramedics.

If you have the symptoms of heart attack, don't drive yourself to the hospital and don't avoid calling for help because you aren't certain the pains you feel are a heart attack. You're in no position to diagnose your symptoms, and no one expects you to. If there was ever a situation where the old 'better safe than sorry' expression applies, this is it. Be sensible. Get medical attention immediately.

Women, the Menopause and Heart Disease

Now that you know what heart disease is, you might be wondering why you need to be concerned about it now. After all, if you're just entering the perimenopause, you're probably in your 40s, or if you've just experienced menopause, you might be in your early 50s.

You're far from being some old-timer who needs to worry about a failing heart – right?

Actually, you're right about the first part of that statement, but wrong about the last. At forty or fifty, you're far from being an old-timer, but heart disease doesn't strike only the elderly. Heart disease is a major killer of women of 50 and over.

Women in their childbearing years are statistically less prone to heart disease than are men of the same age. Your risk of heart disease increases when you reach the menopause, then just keeps on increasing. If your menopause occurs naturally, the risk rises slowly. But if the menopause results from surgery, the risks can rise dramatically and quickly.

What's the Menopause Got to Do with It?

If women have less risk of heart disease before the menopause than do men of the same age, with the same contributing risk factors, why does their postmenopausal risk surpass that of men? To understand this surge in risk, it's important to understand some of the root causes of heart disease in any individual. Although later sections of this chapter discuss these risk factors in detail, one of the most important contributors to heart disease is high blood cholesterol levels. When you develop high blood cholesterol levels, you have too much artery-clogging fat in your bloodstream. The diminished supply of oestrogen that occurs with the menopause, weight gain and the ageing of your cardiovascular system all contribute to developing high cholesterol levels.

Does HRT Lower Your Risk?

A number of medical researchers and scientists believe that a woman's own natural oestrogen might help protect her from heart disease, but they're still studying how the hormone may have that effect. Oestrogen plays an important role in maintaining healthy, strong muscle tissue, including the muscle of the heart. It also has an impact on the blood's level of triglycerides and low-density lipoproteins (LDL) or 'bad' cholesterol, both of which can contribute to atherosclerosis and heart attack. Some studies have shown that oestrogen contributes to healthy, reactive arteries and an increased blood flow. As a result, blood vessels are better able to relax and respond to exercise and physical stress by dilating and providing more blood flow when needed.

Does that mean that you can avoid heart disease through hormone replacement therapies? HRT does have a positive effect on several risk factors for heart disease and stroke. For example, oral forms of HRT increase the level of HDL cholesterol and lower the level of LDL cholesterol. Oestrogen administered in the form of a skin patch also has some beneficial effects on your lipid profile, although it may take longer for these benefits to show up on your blood tests. Even so, doctors don't advise using HRT as a replacement for cholesterol-lowering drugs if you're battling high blood cholesterol levels.

One 25-year-long study in the USA, known as the Harvard Nurses' Health Study, linked HRT with a lower risk of death from heart disease – a benefit that lasted even after ten years of hormone treatment. Another study, the Heart and Oestrogen-Progestin Replacement Study, focused on postmenopausal women who already had coronary heart disease. After approximately four years of follow-up, that study indicated that HRT did not reduce the participants' overall risk of heart attack or death from coronary heart disease as much as previously expected, nor did it have any major impact on their overall risk of stroke. Partial results of a new, ongoing study actually found a small but increased risk of non-fatal heart attack, stroke, deep vein blood clot and pulmonary embolus in women taking one form of HRT for several years. There has been no increased risk in women taking oestrogen alone so far.

Studies continue and you can expect new developments in our understanding of the role of oestrogen, hormone replacement and heart disease in women. Medical experts continue to try to assimilate the results of numerous studies, but this process can be difficult due to differences in the populations of women who entered the studies and the studies' criteria. For now, you need to weigh the potential benefits and risks of any treatment for heart disease, and discuss them carefully with your doctor. (See Chapter 11.)

Heart Disease Risk Factors

As with most killers, heart disease is rarely the product of a single event or condition. Heart disease has long been the focus of intense medical study, contributing to the knowledge about the many illnesses and conditions that can contribute to its development. Some risk factors are yours for life – risks associated with your age, sex, race and genetic inheritance – so you have to construct your healthy life plan with the idea that those risks will always be present. Fortunately, the majority of factors that promote heart disease are controllable. The following sections take a closer look at all of these risk factors – whether they're the products of fate or folly.

The Risk Factors You Own

The key risk factors for developing heart disease that cannot be controlled are few. Women face two unchangeable risks for developing heart disease:

Growing older: The older you get, the greater your risk of developing heart disease. Four out of five people who die of it are 65 or older. And the older women are when they suffer a heart attack, the more likely they are to die of it.

Heredity: If your parents had heart disease, you're more likely to develop it. Sometimes this is because of a propensity to high cholesterol levels. Race-associated conditions can have an impact on heart disease risk, as well. Because the Afro-Caribbean populations can have more severe high blood pressure, they have an elevated risk for developing coronary heart disease.

Having these unchangeable risk factors doesn't mean you're destined to suffer from heart disease. But it does mean that you need to be extra vigilant about controlling the risks you can change.

High Cholesterol

High blood cholesterol is a major risk factor for developing heart disease. After the menopause, women tend to develop high levels of triglycerides (a form of fat) in addition to high levels of low-density lipoprotein (LDL), cholesterol. At the same time, their levels of high-density lipoprotein (HDL) can diminish. All of these factors lead to out-of-balance blood cholesterol levels, too much fat in the bloodstream and the build-up of artery-clogging plaque in the pathways that channel oxygen-rich blood to the heart and brain. For every 1 per cent reduction in elevated blood cholesterol levels, you get a 2 to 3 per cent reduction in your chances of having a heart attack.

Don't misunderstand the issue about cholesterol; cholesterol is a natural, essential substance in the bloodstream. The fraction of your total cholesterol that is HDL cholesterol is actually a protein that helps keep all fats and cholesterols moving through your bloodstream (and not glued to your arterial walls), so it actually helps you stave off a potential heart attack. LDL cholesterol moves cholesterol through the rest of your body – but it also has a tendency to linger in your arteries and stick to the walls. Elevated levels of triglycerides may or may not indicate that you're heading for a heart attack, but as another type of fat in the bloodstream, their levels need to be monitored.

So how much is too much (or not enough) of these substances? Your total blood cholesterol should be under 5.2 millimols per litre (mmol/l), and anything above this is unhealthy.

There are two main types of cholesterol: low-density lipoproteins (LDL), which transport cholesterol from the liver to the cells; and high-density lipoproteins (HDL), which return excess cholesterol back to the liver. Blood lipids is a general term for all the fatty substances in the circulation, including HDL and LDL cholesterol and triglycerides.

The cause of coronary heart disease is a narrowing of the arteries that supply the heart from a gradual accumulation of fatty material, a condition known as atherosclerosis.

Atherosclerosis occurs when LDL cholesterol is deposited on the walls of the coronary arteries, although HDL removes this cholesterol from the circulation and protects against coronary heart disease. The ratio of HDL to LDL is therefore very important, and everyone should aim for a low level of LDL and a high level of HDL.

Although some research has indicated that high cholesterol levels in some people might be a result of heredity, a low-fat diet and regular exercise can help most people maintain healthy blood cholesterol levels. Where those efforts fall short, a variety of cholesterol-lowering drugs, called statins, have entered the market over the past several years. Recent studies have shown that these drugs do actually reduce your risk of dying from heart disease. Although some of these drugs may have side effects, the medications currently on the market are considered safe and effective. Consult your doctor; do not rely on a homeopath or other alternative health care if your lipid profile is abnormal.

Triglycerides are a type of fat found in the blood, but more appealing types of this fat include butter, margarine and vegetable oil. Eating these fats doesn't automatically result in high triglyceride blood levels, however; the partners in crime here seem to be overindulging in alcohol, being overweight or having diabetes.

The effectiveness of HRT in managing blood cholesterol is still the subject of much medical research. Oestrogen has been shown to reduce total blood cholesterol levels and to raise levels of HDL. However, recent studies indicate that some types of oestrogen may actually slightly increase levels of triglycerides in the bloodstream. Your triglycerides may decrease if the oestrogen in your prescription regimen is combined with just the right progestogen for HRT.

High Blood Pressure

High blood pressure (hypertension) is another silent plague of women aged 55 and over. More than half of all women in that age group have blood pressure greater than 140/85 (the high-blood-pressure threshold), but few of them feel its effects. According to the Blood Pressure Association, high blood pressure affects over 16 million people in the

UK. The higher your blood pressure, the greater your risk of stroke, heart attack and heart failure.

Nearly a third of those individuals with high blood pressure are unaware of their condition. Even if you have had normal blood pressure all your life, you might develop high blood pressure after the menopause. And having high blood pressure makes you a prime candidate for developing heart disease. High blood pressure also contributes to kidney disease and can lead to congestive heart failure, heart attack and stroke.

As with cholesterol, everyone needs blood pressure. After all, blood pressure results from the force of your heart pumping your blood through your veins. If you exercise or become excited, your heart rate increases, sending more blood through your system. If your arteries are clean and wide open, the blood flows freely; if they're narrow or blocked, the build-up of blood trying to course through your veins puts pressure on the arterial walls – and that's high blood pressure. If your arteries are clean and healthy, your blood pressure rises for a short period of time, then returns to normal as the blood moves through your circulatory system.

If you have hypertension, however, your blood pressure is greater than 140/85, even when you're at rest; the extra pressure on your heart and arteries never lets up. If high blood pressure occurs in a person with atherosclerosis, the walls of the vessels are toughened and less elastic, and even less able to cope with stress.

High blood pressure is a particular threat to people of Afro-Caribbean origin, women over 35, heavy drinkers, obese women and those with diabetes or kidney disease. However, a family history of high blood pressure isn't a strong risk indicator – one inheritance you can be happy to forget about.

Most doctors consider 120/80 the ideal blood pressure reading. Although some people have suffered from low blood pressure, it's a relatively uncommon occurrence and not life-threatening. Regular exercise and a diet high in vegetables and fruit, but low in sodium, can help control high blood pressure. If diet, exercise and weight loss (when indicated) don't bring blood pressure down, your doctor may prescribe drug therapy.

Diabetes

Diabetes is another heart disease risk factor that is of particular concern to women. Women who have diabetes are at a significantly greater risk of developing heart disease than non-diabetic women. Having diabetes ups your risk of heart disease and stroke by two to four times.

Diabetes mellitus occurs when the body is unable to produce adequate amounts of insulin or efficiently use the insulin it produces (insulin resistance). Insulin is produced in the pancreas, and the body uses it to process the sugar and carbohydrates you consume into energy. Type 2, or adult onset, diabetes is the most common form of the disease, and this usually occurs at middle age. Symptoms of diabetes include weight loss, blurred vision, intense thirst, fatigue, excessive urination and hunger. Doctors test for diabetes through assessing the level of glucose (sugar) in your blood. If a random (non-fasting) glucose screening test is borderline or abnormal, or if your family history is very strong, the doctor may decide to repeat the test. In that test, the doctor may ask you to fast before the first blood sample is taken; then, after you drink a specifically prepared glucose solution, blood samples are taken again at two one-hour intervals. If two of the samples show an elevated blood glucose level, you're considered to be diabetic.

Doctors don't know what causes the development of diabetes, and no drug can cure it. However, diabetes can be controlled – and sometimes disappears altogether – through diet, exercise and weight loss. Statistics show that 80 to 90 per cent of people with Type 2 diabetes are overweight, and many have high blood pressure and/or lead inactive lives. Although a large number of diabetics require insulin or drug therapy, many others are able to control their disease through behaviour modification, such as diet, exercise and weight loss – a lifelong change that offers big rewards.

Obesity

Few diseases are as common and as potentially damaging (both emotionally and physically) as obesity. In fact, obesity has never been more common; the numbers of obese people in the UK continue to rise at alarming levels. More than half of adult Britons are overweight or obese, conditions defined in general by a body weight more than 30 per cent over the ideal for the body's height and frame, or having an abnormally high body mass index (BMI). Obesity is damaging in ways few non-obese people can imagine; unlike most other diseases, obesity is commonly viewed as a disease of weakness, self-indulgence and laziness. Obese people often are the object of ridicule and disdain. Unlike other heart disease risk factors, obesity is plainly visible.

The link between hypertension (high blood pressure) and obesity is particularly strong. It is estimated that over 75 per cent of all diagnosed hypertension is directly related to obesity.

Although obesity can result in obvious emotional distress, its health-damaging effects are even more insidious. Obesity is strongly linked to heart disease in ways that are still under study, but some research indicates that nearly 70 per cent of diagnosed cases of heart disease may be directly linked to obesity. And obesity is a gateway disease for numerous other conditions, including diabetes, high blood pressure, high blood cholesterol levels, kidney disease, sleep apnoea, depression, menstrual irregularities, joint disease and even some forms of cancer.

Although weight gain in middle age isn't uncommon for both men and women, women are at special risk for heart disease from their postmenopausal weight gain. The reason is the location of the added weight; many women tend to add weight in their abdomen and upper body during the menopause. This type of fat seems to be linked very closely with a number of other risk factors for heart disease, including diabetes. And at middle-age, women are particularly susceptible to weight gain. The body's metabolism begins to slow down during the perimenopause; as a result, the body burns fewer calories, even at rest. So if a middle-aged woman continues to consume the same number of calories that she consumed in her youth, the chances are good that she will gain weight.

Body mass index (BMI) is used to calculate both overweight and obesity, while height and weight tables offer another option for determining obesity. Calculate your own BMI by dividing your weight in kilos by your height in metres squared, for example 82kg/1.72 x 1.72 = BMI 29; or visit the British Nutrition Foundation website (*www.nutrition.org.uk*) for information on diet and an automatic BMI calculator.

Although so many Western people suffer from obesity, researchers are still trying to determine all the factors that contribute to it. Some contributors are controllable – things such as leading a sedentary lifestyle and consuming a high-fat, high-calorie diet. But if those factors were the only causes of obesity, fewer individuals would suffer from the disease. In fact, our sex, age, individual biological and genetic make-up, psychological condition and environment each appear capable of playing a major role in the development of obesity.

Still, behaviour modification is a powerful weapon against obesity. A low-calorie, low-fat, high-fibre diet and regular exercise are the first line of defence against this disease. But for many people, other methods prove helpful, including drug therapy, psychotherapy, hypnosis, acupuncture and even surgery. As this disease continues to become more prevalent in our society, look for further discoveries and advancement in its treatment.

Smoking

Smoking tobacco is hard on your entire body, but it delivers a particularly hard blow to your heart. Each time you draw in a lungful of tobacco smoke, you temporarily increase your heart rate and blood pressure and deplete the oxygen in your bloodstream that should be going to feed your heart and other body tissues. If you smoke even one to four cigarettes a day, you're doubling your chances of having a heart attack – and very few smokers smoke four or fewer cigarettes in the average day. Smoke a pack or more, and your risk goes up four times. Over 30 per cent of all deaths due to coronary heart disease are attributable to smoking. There's little disagreement in the healthcare profession about the dangers of tobacco addiction. Smoking is linked to innumerable other diseases and conditions, including a wide range of cardiovascular and other heart diseases, chronic lung diseases, and many forms of cancer. There are 31,820 deaths per year in the UK due to smoking. If you smoke 25 cigarettes a day, you are 25 times more likely to die from lung cancer than a non-smoker.

But hey – you knew all of that, didn't you? And, you undoubtedly know that smoking-related diseases are incredibly preventable. Not only do even long-time smokers experience very immediate benefits from stopping, but also smokers who have already developed tobacco smoking-related diseases can benefit from kicking the habit. Your body begins repairing smoke-related damage within an hour after your last cigarette.

Although not all the studies have included women, some have shown that men who stop smoking can have the same risk of heart disease as nonsmokers within three to five years of stopping. If you're a smoker, the best thing you can do for your heart (and the rest of your body, for that matter) is to stop smoking now.

The British Medical Association has conservatively estimated that passive smoking causes 1,000 deaths a year, but the figure is likely to be far higher. In fact, research at Imperial College London suggests that 3,600 people a year die as a result of exposure to secondhand smoke at home, with a further 700 a year from exposure at work.

Smoking is an extremely addictive habit, however, that hooks users physically, psychologically and emotionally. If you can't just throw away the packet and stop smoking, you're in the majority; talk to your doctor about smoking cessation programmes, nicotine replacement therapy and other techniques that can help you kick the habit. If you have children, remind yourself of how important you are to them as a role model; your stopping smoking may help them decide not to start.

Controlling Your Risks

As you've probably determined by reading the previous sections on individual risk factors for developing heart disease, you actually can exercise (get it?) a great deal of control over your personal susceptibility to this disease and the conditions that contribute to it. Although you might have a genetic susceptibility to high blood pressure, high cholesterol or diabetes, or your age itself may increase your chances of contracting heart disease, you can take positive action to manage your overall risks. Here are some suggestions:

· **Eat a low-fat, low-cholesterol, high-fibre diet.** The less saturated fat you consume, the better you'll be able to manage blood cholesterol levels. Try to build your diet around fresh fruits, vegetables and whole grains. Limit the amount of animal fat, meat and dairy products you consume, and go easy on the salt – especially if you suffer from high blood pressure. And eat some soya; eating 25 grams of soya protein – from soya milk, veggieburgers or tofu – a day can help lower your LDL cholesterol level by as much as 5 to 10 per cent. (For more information about the benefits and sources of soya, see Chapter 13.)

· **Manage your weight.** Ask your GP to help you determine what your weight should be and how you can best reach and maintain that weight. The first step to weight management is diet management. Eat a low-calorie, low-fat diet, and weigh yourself regularly. To check the kinds and amounts of foods you eat, keep a food diary of your meals, including calorie and fat gram count. No matter what other lifestyle changes you make, being overweight or obese can dramatically increase your risks of suffering from some form of heart disease.

· **Exercise regularly.** Physical activity not only helps control obesity, but also helps dramatically reduce the severity of many conditions that contribute to heart disease. And the really good news about exercise is that you can get it in just about any way you like. Walking, hoovering the floor, taking stairs instead of lifts, and dancing are all great ways to up your activity level. Doctors advise taking at least 30 minutes of exercise at least three days a week, but an hour of exercise four days a week is better. Your exercise should boost your heart rate, but it doesn't have to be a 'killer' routine. Try to combine both weight training (such as lifting weights) and aerobic (swimming, walking, running) exercises, preceded and followed by a series of stretching movements in your routine.

· **Drink alcohol in moderation.** If you drink alcohol, keep your consumption to no more than one drink a day.

· **Stop smoking.** Now – use whatever means necessary.

· **Find ways to avoid or relieve stress.** Being stressed out is not only unpleasant but also hard on your heart. When you're under stress, your heart rate can go up, your breathing can become shallow and all your muscles can become tense. If you want your heart and brain to be nourished by a strong, healthy flow of oxygenated blood, learn to keep stress to a minimum. Exercise helps, as does relaxation therapy, meditation and quiet time spent enjoying the things you love.

CHAPTER 8

Maintaining Bone Health

Osteoporosis is a threat that every woman should take seriously, and that threat grows even more serious as the menopause approaches. Your best defence against osteoporosis is to understand your risks for developing this disease and to follow a sensible plan for minimizing those risks and protecting your bones – for the rest of your life.

Close-up on Osteoporosis

Osteoporosis is a degenerative bone disease that every woman should view as a potential enemy. An estimated 3 million people in the UK suffer from osteoporosis. The condition affects one in three women and one in 12 men and causes 200,000 bone breaks a year and 40 deaths a day.

If your first instinct upon reading these statistics is to dash out and stock up on calcium supplements, hold on a minute. Your best weapon against osteoporosis is knowledge; take a moment to get the facts on this disease. Then, you can get the calcium supplements – and follow the simple prescription for bone health offered later in this chapter.

There are big differences between people in the rate at which they lose calcium. Women are at particular risk after the menopause because the fall in female hormone levels weakens the bones over a period of years. In the UK, bone density testing (densitometry) is done as a form of screening. It should be carried out on anyone over 65, and may be advised earlier if you have an early menopause or hysterectomy, absence of periods or known low female hormone levels, or a family history of osteoporosis.

What Is Osteoporosis?

Osteoporosis is a disease in which your bones lose density. When you have osteoporosis, your bone tissue deteriorates, leaving your bones structurally weak and susceptible to fractures. Typically, victims of osteoporosis suffer fractures in their hips, spinal vertebrae and wrists, but any bone in the body can crumble when this disease progresses to an advanced state.

Many people think of their adult bones as a stable and unchanging support for the growing, vital parts of the body's make-up. But bones are alive. Bone tissue is in a constant state of evolution, as the body replaces old bone cells with new bone cells. When you're a child, your bones have a lot of growing to do, so your body produces much more new bone than it takes back in through reabsorption (the process of absorbing old bone cells back into the body).

But at around the age of 30, your body reaches a stage of peak bone mass, where your bones are as large and dense as they will ever be. At that stage, reabsorption slowly begins to outpace bone production. If reabsorption becomes too rapid or if bone cell production becomes too slow, you're at risk of developing osteoporosis. If you didn't build your bones to their optimum size during the years leading to peak bone mass, your risk is even greater.

Young girls need to build bone density, but it's not a subject that interests most teenagers. So if you have a young daughter or niece, make sure she's taking in adequate amounts of calcium, especially during her early teenage years' growth spurt.

At time of writing, there is no cure for osteoporosis. But you can slow the progress of the disease dramatically through a treatment plan involving some combination of medication, diet and exercise. Recent experiments with drugs that may actually help rebuild lost bone tissue offer true encouragement to victims of this disease and those who treat them. But remember, prevention is easier than treatment.

How Osteoporosis Strikes

Osteoporosis, even today, is underdiagnosed and undertreated. As with many deadly diseases, osteoporosis gains much of its power through its ability to progress silently without any readily apparent signs or symptoms. Bone tissue loss isn't painful in its early stages – everyone experiences it every day. Weak bones don't ache or creak or exhibit any other kind of warning. In fact, osteoporosis frequently is diagnosed only after someone suffers a bone fracture. And even then, if the person who suffered the break and/or her doctor doesn't suspect that the break could be related to osteoporosis, and follow up with the proper diagnostic tests, the disease can remain undiagnosed and untreated.

Osteoporotic bones lose mass very slowly; over a period of time, the bones become so fragile that they can break under very slight strain. Every year, osteoporosis is responsible for:

· 70,000 hip fractures
· 120,000 vertebral fractures
· 50,000 wrist fractures

Some of these figures may be underestimates, since certain fractures aren't even recognized when they occur. The pain resulting from crumbled vertebrae might seem like a back strain, for example. If the broken bone goes unnoticed or the break is apparent but no one connects it to the disease, osteoporosis continues to erode the bones until another fracture occurs. By the time the warning flag goes up, the disease may have advanced to a critical stage.

Ninety per cent of all hip fractures are associated with osteoporosis and result from a fall. Most falls happen to women in their homes in the afternoon. When your legs lose strength, your eyesight becomes weaker (especially your peripheral vision) and your balance and flexibility diminish, you're more likely to fall and be unable to catch yourself. These changes can begin in your 40s and 50s, making osteoporosis a real concern to you now.

Diagnosing the Disease

Besides warning you about osteoporosis before you suffer a fracture, bone density tests can help you determine your rate of bone loss and help you gauge the effectiveness of your efforts to slow that loss. A bone density test can tell you how your bone density compares to that of healthy bone tissue from a person of your age and – more importantly – to that of an average 25-year-old.

Fractures from minor accidents can indicate bone loss. If you have suffered a fracture after a minor fall, you should ask your doctor about conducting a bone density test. Other late signs of osteoporosis occur in many women aged 65 and older, including stooped shoulders or a loss of height.

The Menopause and Osteoporosis

As you've learned, women make up the vast majority of those diagnosed with osteoporosis. As you approach menopause, your chances of developing this disease increase dramatically. Here's why: your bones are in a constant state of remodelling its bone tissue, by removing old bone tissue cells through reabsorption and creating new ones. However, as with many remodellers, the body is more adept at tearing down the old than at building the new. Your body depends upon its growth hormones – especially oestrogen – to help pace the remodelling process.

Oestrogen Loss Depletes Bone Tissue

So what role does oestrogen play in this whole remodelling process? Oestrogen protects your bones by controlling the amount of bone removed by reabsorption. When your oestrogen levels drop after the menopause (either gradually through natural menopause or dramatically as a result of induced menopause), your bones lose that protection. As a result of this, in the five to eight years following the menopause, your bone loss can increase dramatically as your body adjusts to the loss of ovarian oestrogen.

If you've gone through an early menopause, your body has endured a greater-than-normal oestrogen loss and your risk of experiencing accelerated bone loss increases. And if you've ever experienced extensive or frequent bouts of amenorrhoea (lack of periods), your bones have been through periods of accelerated bone loss due to a loss of oestrogen protection.

Your parathyroid gland secretes a hormone that controls the amount of calcium released by your bones into the bloodstream. If this gland becomes overactive (hyperparathyroidism), your bones can release too much calcium and contribute to the development of osteoporosis. This condition is particularly dangerous for women in the menopause. The good news, however, is that hyperparathyroidism is a treatable condition.

The Facts about Postmenopausal Bone Loss

Although your bone loss is gradual in the years between achieving peak bone mass and entering the menopause, after the menopause the loss increases dramatically. The average woman loses up to 3 per cent of bone mass a year after the menopause. So women can lose up to 20 per cent of their bone mass in the first five to seven years following the menopause.

So does that mean that every woman emerges from the first decade of the menopause with thin, fragile bones? Certainly not! Remember that the condition of your bones plays a role in preserving their mass, as do a number of other factors, including heredity, environment, diet and exercise.

All of these facts lead to only one logical conclusion: every woman – regardless of her age or health – needs to understand her risks for developing osteoporosis and to have a sound, ongoing plan for maintaining her bone health. Waiting until you're older or until you've entered the menopause to protect yourself against osteoporosis just won't work; by then, you could already be losing the battle against bone loss.

Understanding and Controlling Your Risks

If every woman goes through the menopause, why doesn't every woman develop osteoporosis? The risk factors for developing this disease go well beyond age and hormonal production rates. Here are some of the genetic, environmental and other risk factors of developing this disease:

· **Body make-up:** Women with thin, small frames are at greater risk of suffering excessive bone loss as they age.

- **A family history of osteoporosis:** If other women (or men) in your family developed this disease, your risk for developing it goes up.
- **Caucasian or Asian race:** Afro-Caribbean women have a much lower incidence of postmenopausal osteoporosis than do Northern European and Asian women. However, they still need the same screening for other risk factors.
- **Taking certain medications:** If you've taken steroids (such as prednisone), anticonvulsants, thyroid hormone replacement therapy or lithium for more than three months, your risks of developing osteoporosis increase.
- **Eating disorders:** A history of eating disorders such as anorexia or bulimia can increase your risks. Infrequent or irregular periods can be a sign that excessive dieting is resulting in low oestrogen levels.
- **Lifestyle choices:** Excess consumption of alcohol, inadequate calcium intake, tobacco smoking and a lack of exercise all can contribute to the development of osteoporosis over time. If your diet is low in calcium, you're putting yourself at risk of developing the disease.

As you can see, some risk factors are controllable and others aren't. But you have many options available to you for preventing or slowing the progress of osteoporosis. The National Osteoporosis Society recommends these three steps for preventing or managing the disease:

- Eat a healthy diet that includes ample supplies of calcium and vitamin D.
- Incorporate weight-bearing exercise, such as walking or weightlifting, in your regular exercise plan (and that means doing these exercises three or more times a week).
- Stop smoking, and don't overindulge in alcohol.

Eating for Strong Bones

You already know that your diet plays a big role in your overall health, but a balanced diet rich in calcium and vitamin D is particularly important for preventing or slowing the progress of osteoporosis. Your body stores kilograms of calcium in its bones, and calcium is an essential nutrient for all of your body's organs and tissues. Maintaining your calcium levels helps keep all of your body – not just its bones – healthy and fit.

A woman's calcium requirement changes as she ages. Between the ages of 11 and 24, you should get at least 1,200 milligrams of calcium every day. You can drop that amount to 800 milligrams per day from the of 25 to 50. By the time you reach 50, you need at least 1,200 to 1,500 milligrams of calcium every day. (If you're still having periods or taking oestrogen, the lower number will do, but if you're in the menopause and not on oestrogen, move up to the higher amount.) What foods give you the greatest calcium boost? Here are just some examples (remember to check food product labels):

FOOD	MILLIGRAMS OF CALCIUM
Fruit yogurt, 100g	160
Edam cheese, 100g	770
Skimmed milk, 190ml	235
Semi-skimmed milk, 190ml	231
Sardines, tinned with bones, 100g	550
Figs, dried, 100g	250
Kale, cooked, 100g	150
Spinach, fresh or cooked, 100g	160
Macaroni cheese, 100g	170
Tofu, steamed, 100g	510
Vanilla ice cream, dairy, 100g	130
Cheddar cheese, 100g	720

But getting plenty of calcium isn't your only dietary weapon against osteoporosis. Vitamin D doesn't put more calcium into your system, but it does help your body use the calcium you eat. Your body absorbs vitamin D from the sun; if you live in a cold or northern climate, or don't spend much time outdoors, vitamin D added to your calcium supplement will help your gastrointestinal system absorb the calcium. Women between the ages of 51 and 70 need about 400 units of vitamin D every day. Eggs and some fish, including sardines, mackerel and herring, contain small amounts of vitamin D.

Don't misunderstand: eating a well-balanced diet with adequate amounts of calcium and vitamin D won't guarantee an osteoporosis-free life. But without question it's the best method available for helping your body prevent or slow the disease.

Can you be a vegetarian and eat a bone-healthy diet?
Yes you can! However, you must eat a well-balanced diet of beans, seeds, grains and a broad variety of vegetables. Some vegetarians eat eggs and dairy products, and therefore have more access to calcium in their diet. If you eat no dairy products at all, you need to carefully monitor your calcium intake and consider taking supplements.

Using Calcium and Vitamin Supplements

Although diet is always the best source of vitamins and nutrients, as you approach the menopause, you may find that your diet needs some boosters in the form of supplements. Some estimates indicate that most menopausal women eat only about half as much calcium as they require each day. And many women have trouble digesting dairy products, so upping their intake of milk, yogurt and cheese may not be an option for getting the increased calcium their bones demand.

Calcium supplements are available in a number of forms today, and they can be a great benefit to any woman approaching the menopause. Bear these facts in mind when choosing and using calcium supplements:

- The elemental calcium content of any supplement is what matters most. Check the label carefully to make sure the supplement carries the appropriate amount of elemental calcium.
- Choose calcium supplements from reputable makers; check the label to see if the calcium is purified and look for any guarantees of the reliability of the source.
- Calcium works best when you take it in 500 milligram doses, divided over the course of the day.

Your body may be intolerant of a fast, sizeable increase of calcium; signs of that intolerance can be indigestion or wind. Try to build slowly towards your full dosage, and if your system continues to have problems, try a different calcium supplement. A calcium-supplemented orange juice may reduce these side effects.

Because vitamin D is available in few non-dairy foods, many people need to supplement their daily supply. Most all-purpose vitamins contain a daily dose of vitamin D, as do some calcium supplements. And minerals such as phosphorous and magnesium are important for bone health, too. Again, adequate doses of these are available in most multivitamins.

Remember, a well-balanced diet is always your best source of nutrients, including vitamins and minerals. But as women approach the menopause, most find that they need supplements to round out their daily requirements of calcium. As with any health-related plan, however, discuss all dietary and food supplement decisions with your doctor before making any changes in your current practices.

Exercising as Prevention

You probably didn't hear it here first, but exercise is an absolute must for a healthy life – and a healthy passage through the menopause. Exercise plays a particularly important role in protecting your bones. Studies have shown that weight-bearing exercise builds strong, healthy, resilient bones and can slow the progress of bone loss. Walking, one of the most popular forms of exercise, seems to be particularly helpful in encouraging new bone growth. Exercise not only helps maintain your bones' health but also keeps your joints and muscles flexible and strong. Those improvements alone go a long way toward helping you prevent fractures caused by falls.

Most health-care professionals recommend 30 minutes of weight-bearing exercise – such as walking or other moderately intense physical activity – three days a week, as part of a total exercise programme that also includes aerobic and stretching exercises. If you go for a weightlifting programme, make sure you get the help and advice of your doctor in planning a programme that will offer you the maximum benefit and the minimum risk of strain or injury.

Exercise alone won't prevent osteoporosis. But if you combine a sensible exercise programme with a well-balanced diet (remember those high levels of calcium and vitamin D) and avoid smoking and excess alcohol consumption, you'll go a long way to preserving your bone health, even after the menopause.

Using SERMs or HRT for Bone Health

Diet, exercise and nutritional supplements can all slow the bone loss your body experiences after the menopause, but they can't stop it. However, most doctors agree that oestrogen therapy can halt bone loss during this time and may actually contribute to bone growth.

Selective estrogen receptor modulators (SERMs) are drugs that act in a similar way to oestrogen on the bone, helping to maintain bone density and reduce fracture rates, specifically at the spine.

Hormone replacement therapy (HRT) is oestrogen replacement for women at the menopause, which help maintain bone density and reduce fracture rates for the duration of therapy.

fact

Calcitonin is a hormone produced naturally by cells in the thyroid gland. It plays a part in regulating the formation and breakdown of bone. Synthetic calcitonin (derived from salmon) has the same effects as the human hormone and is used to prevent bone breakdown. It is given by injection or nasal spray.

SERMs are a relatively new class of drugs that prevent bone loss. Early tests have shown that SERMs increase bone mass and, after three years of use, can reduce the risk of spine fractures by about 50 per cent.

Whether you choose to use natural oestrogens or 'designer' oestrogens to prevent postmenopausal bone loss, your doctor is your best source of advice and information for making this important decision. But don't depend on either approach as your only solution for staving off bone loss. No matter what type of medications or supplements you take, a healthy diet and regular weight-bearing exercise are important components of your anti-osteoporosis arsenal.

CHAPTER 9

The Menopause and Sexuality

Women in the perimenopause can be surprised to find their sexual appetites changing. The reasons for shifts in sexual readiness and desire are as complex as human sexuality itself, and include physical, emotional, psychological and chemical changes natural in a maturing body. By learning more about the potential impact of the menopause on your own sexuality, you're better prepared to manage your experience.

A New Sexual Revolution

Popular culture is woven together by an infinite public appetite for sexuality; if you doubt this, just count the number of sexual references you encounter in any evening spent watching television, reading magazines, watching films or listening to commercial radio. Nevertheless, the public fascination with female sexuality has very definite boundaries, and those boundaries are determined by age. So while the sexual appetites and capabilities of women in their 20s and 30s seem to hold endless fascination for the public at large, that interest flags dramatically when the subject turns to the sex life of women in the menopause. And when you do see or hear popular references to the sexuality of the over-40 female set, those references are more likely intended to disturb or amuse – not titillate – the viewer or listener.

In the past, many people assumed that women lost their desire for sex as they approached the menopause, and that the passage through the menopause led inevitably toward the eventual death of the libido. Today, most people know that idea is simply untrue and dismiss it as outdated mythology; still, not everyone understands all of the ways the physical changes of the menopause can affect sexuality.

A landmark 1986 study by Masters & Johnson (*Sex and Ageing – Expectations and Reality*) found that women can remain sexually active through their entire lives with no decline in orgasmic potential, and may become more orgasmic. The study also found that normal changes of sexual response and ageing don't equate to decreased sexual functioning.

Thanks to the burgeoning numbers of women moving into midlife today, however, the discussion, research and medical information on maturing female sexuality has never been richer. Talking about libido with other people is no longer considered taboo. Women can turn to doctors, health-care professionals and books such as this one to educate themselves about exactly what kinds of physical symptoms and changes may affect their sexuality during the menopause, and how to maintain optimum sexual health during this time. That understanding paves the way for a sexual revolution as socially significant as the first one these Baby Boomers experienced back in the 1960s and 1970s – an era of the sexually confident, healthy and vital midlife woman!

The Physical Facts of Life

If you abandon the idea that sexual problems of midlife are all in the head, the next step toward managing your own maturing sexual health is to understand the facts of life for this stage of your life. So what physical symptoms and changes can interfere with sexual desire and pleasure as the menopause approaches? Here are the most common:

· Vaginal dryness
· Pain during penetration
· Reduced response to clitoral stimulation and other sexual stimuli

Some of these changes are absolutely normal parts of the ageing process and don't represent alarming signals that sexual life is drawing to a close. Women (and men, for that matter) typically experience a slowdown in their biological sexual response. Women may take longer to become aroused, for example, and some women report that they have fewer orgasmic contractions and shorter orgasms in general. These changes just mean that lovemaking takes on a new schedule or some new practices – changes that can benefit lovemaking at any age. Other physical changes are transient and treatable, either with medical hormonal therapies or non-hormonal, natural techniques.

But a maturing woman can undergo a number of physical and medical events that can trigger the symptoms and conditions of flagging sexual health as well. These events include:

· Illnesses, both physical and emotional, including (but not limited to) cardiac problems, hypertension, cancer, bladder disease, depression and arthritis
· Medications used to treat any of the above illnesses, including some antihypertensives, antidepressants, tranquillizers and antihistamines
· Medical treatments, such as radiation therapy, chemotherapy or surgery

Don't get the impression that if you take blood pressure medication or undergo surgery that you're embarking on a life of sexual abstinence. Sexual dysfunction resulting from illness or long-term treatments such as chemotherapy can pass as the illness and treatment side effects fade. A number of alternative medications can replace those that create sexual problems for certain individuals.

> Medical causes of female sexual dysfunction are rarely permanent or untreatable. That's why it's important that any woman experiencing any change in her sexual functions should talk to her doctor. If a medical condition or treatment is contributing to the problem, a health professional can explain how long the problem may persist, or change treatments or medications that may be triggering it.

Hormones and Sexuality

One of the primary causes for many sexual health issues in perimenopausal and menopausal women is the loss of oestrogen that results from the slowdown and eventual cessation of a woman's reproductive cycle. Hormonal imbalances can trigger or exacerbate many of the physical symptoms that can erode a healthy, perimenopausal woman's sex life.

Hormones – especially oestrogen – play an important role in your body's sexual response. Oestrogen helps to nourish all of your body's tissues, including your vagina, vulva and urethra. Oestrogen also helps keep the clitoris well nourished and responsive; with less oestrogen, the clitoris can lose some of its ability to respond to touch.

As your vaginal wall becomes thinner and drier, your vagina can become shorter, narrower and less elastic. In particularly severe cases, sex can then become quite painful. Lack of lubrication and vaginal walls that just won't give can also make sex less appealing – both to the woman and her partner.

A lack of oestrogen will also result in a change in the normal vaginal pH and lower levels of lactobacillus, the normal bacteria that helps ward off most vaginal infections in reproductive-age women. Thus, if your vagina goes through marked changes in pH levels, you may find that you're more susceptible to vaginal infections. These infections can make your vagina feel raw and irritated, create abnormal vaginal discharge and make sexual intercourse a painful, burning experience. Oestrogen replacement therapy can improve vaginal secretions and tone, and can even be used in the form of a vaginal cream for more rapid effects. (Other techniques for maintaining vaginal health are found in 'Maintaining Your Sexual Health', later in this chapter.)

Hormones play another critical role in strengthening or diminishing the libido; the sex hormones – oestrogen and progesterone – contribute to mood. If you grow anxious, depressed, irritable or exhausted as a result of hormone deficiencies, your sex life can suffer.

Beyond the Physical Factor

Without question, a woman's psychological and emotional state can trigger many of the physical symptoms associated with ageing sexuality. When a woman has low self-esteem or a poor body image, for example, she can have a greatly reduced response to stimulation. Anxiety, sleeplessness and hot flushes can interfere with a woman's ability to anticipate or enjoy sex and contribute to one or more of the previously listed physical symptoms. Decreased sexual activity itself can lead to diminished sexual desire, pleasure and response. A woman with a sexually dysfunctional partner – or no partner at all – can be at risk of losing her own sexual health as a result.

See 'Your Mate May Be Menopausal, Too' in Chapter 1, 'Every Woman's Menopause... and Yours'; 'Changes in Libido' in Chapter 2, 'Understanding the Symptoms of the Perimenopause'; and Chapter 17, 'Finding Your New Sexuality', which discusses techniques for revitalizing your sex drive.

Any woman knows that her most important responses to sexual stimulation take place in her brain; as a result, any number of conditions or illnesses can impair a woman's libido, including alcoholism, fatigue, depression and chronic illnesses. It's hard to dispute the fact that our libido is all tangled up in our self-esteem. Perimenopause and natural menopause are transitions associated with ageing, and if self-esteem suffers as a result of ageing, sexual desire may suffer, too. Our bodies change during the perimenopause; that, too, is an undeniable fact. The degree of that change varies, of course, and we have many tools at our disposal to help maintain our physical health and vitality as we grow older. But women who combat weight gain, fatigue, depression and feelings of isolation during the perimenopause are at risk of suffering from flagging sexual desire as well.

And our partners – male or female – are changing, too. Two women going through the perimenopause at the same time may experience a multitude of sexual issues as they try to maintain their sexual closeness as each rides her own roller coaster of menopausal symptoms. Men can experience a loss of sexual potency and desire as they age, and that can have a direct impact on the sexual confidence and health of their partners. If a sexual partner seems uninterested in sex or unable to sustain an erection or become aroused, it's easy for the other partner to feel inadequate, undesirable and definitely unsexy. It's also not easy to feel good about yourself if your husband or partner decides to dump you for a trophy wife or neglects you to chase after a mistress.

You have an important opportunity to improve your sex life during the perimenopause. This time of transition encourages women to reassess their lives, their relationships and their attitudes towards living. You have a wide variety of physical and psychological tools available to you to help take your sexuality to new heights as your body enjoys sex for reasons that have nothing to do with reproduction.

Maintaining Your Sexual Health

Now, you might read the preceding paragraphs and think, 'I'm doomed to lose my sexuality, because I (along with every other woman living on this planet) have one of these conditions, use some of these medications or am experiencing some of these issues.' But you can throw those fears away right now. Most of the events, issues, treatments and so on listed above can – but may not necessarily – lead to temporary sexual dysfunction. Nearly every symptom or problem that affects your sexual health is treatable, reversible or even avoidable. But, as with any area of your health maintenance, you can't count on someone else – your doctor, friends, therapist or partner – to protect and manage your sexual health. That job is yours.

fact

In a survey of 45- to 65-year-old men and women conducted in 2001 by *Newsweek* magazine in the USA, 30 per cent of women and 34 per cent of men surveyed thought sex was more enjoyable for people their age than for younger people; 40 per cent of women and 47 per cent of men said it was 'about the same', while only 16 per cent and 12 per cent (respectively) thought sex 'less enjoyable' with age.

If you, like the vast majority of men and women in this country, intend to remain sexually active throughout a long and healthy life, what can you do to ensure that you maintain your sexual health through the years ahead? Later chapters talk about specific ideas for exploring and enhancing your new sexuality and for treating causes of sexual dysfunction. Chapters 11 and 12, for example, discuss hormone replacement therapy and its alternatives – common and very effective methods for treating a wide range of physical (and emotional) symptoms that impair sexual response and functions. And Chapter 17 covers the ways you can keep your sex drive alive and happy during and well after the menopause. But before you begin any of those treatment or practise alternatives, you have four very basic tools at your disposal for monitoring and maintaining your sexual health:

- Monitor your sexual health and pay attention to changes in your sexual responses and feelings
- Maintain an open dialogue with your GP about sexual problems and solutions
- Maintain your vaginal health
- Use appropriate birth control methods while in the perimenopause

Listen to Your Sexual Self

One of the most important things you can do to maintain your sexual health is to pay attention to what your body and mind are telling you about your feelings about your sexuality, your attitude toward sex in general, and your evolving sexual response. Your sexuality evolves with the rest of you, and the entire package has changed dramatically over the last 20 years. To illustrate, just choose an answer to this question:

My idea of a great evening is:
a. Dancing and drinking until dawn in a local nightspot
b. Getting picked up in a bar or nightclub
c. Going out on a first date
d. Sitting at home reading, watching television or doing anything else that enables me to wear jogging pants without sweating

Many of those who choose D (and that's many of us over the age of 40), wouldn't have chosen it 20 years ago. And that's not a sign of age – it's a sign of maturity. Your sexual interests and responses change, too; sexual techniques you used to enjoy might have lost some – or all – of their appeal in time. As your sexual tastes evolve, you can find totally new and different ways to enjoy sex, and that's just one of the benefits of ageing.

Don't try to force yourself into a sexuality that doesn't fit; some people have strong libidos and sex drives; others don't. Think about your sexuality and accept the sexual person you are, but don't try to settle for less or berate yourself because you don't want more. Be honest with your sexual self.

But if you suddenly realize that sex no longer holds any interest for you; or that you don't like your body enough to share it in sexual relations with anyone; or that it's just too painful, awkward, difficult or otherwise unpleasant to bother with sex, you need to stop and ask yourself when – and why – these feelings arose in you. You're too young (at any age) to just walk away from a sexually fulfilling life.

If you find your interest in sex or your ability to respond to sexual stimulation fading dramatically, you shouldn't chalk it up to maturity. Enjoying your sexuality is part of leading a healthy, well-rounded life. And a sudden or severe loss of interest in sex can signal other problems – both emotional and physical – that can grow worse as time goes by. Remember, the popular saying 'use it or lose it' can be frequently applied to sexuality. Long periods of abstinence can undermine your ability to become aroused, and lack of sexual activity can promote a diminished response to sexual stimulation.

In any event, you aren't better off just forgetting about it. You deserve and benefit from a healthy, active sexual self – whether you have a partner or not. Even single, older women should be able to feel sexually aroused by certain images – whether it's a good-looking actor, an advertisement for lingerie or a steamy passage in a book. If you aren't enjoying (or even thinking about) sex, you have many options for regaining your sexual enjoyment – whether that involves exploring new sexual techniques, examining your attitudes about your sexuality or investigating possible medical causes for your diminishing sexual interests or abilities.

Let's Talk about S-E-X

As your sexuality matures with you, you might experience any or all of the problems or issues discussed in this chapter. And, in most cases, you may need to talk to a medical professional, therapist or other counsellor or consultant to find the best resolution for those problems. If you aren't comfortable discussing medical or emotional aspects of your sexuality or sexual health, that discomfort can make your situation seem even more frustrating and hopeless. Your ability to talk about issues – ranging from painful intercourse to a lack of response to stimulation – is crucial to establish a trusting relationship with your doctor, and to become comfortable discussing your sexual health with that person.

Talking to a professional can help. If a lack of interest in sex is a side effect of a growing sense of depression and isolation, a counsellor, friend or therapist may be able to help you explore and resolve the source of those feelings. If sex is physically less enjoyable – even painful – a gynaecologist can prescribe medications, exercises or other treatments to resolve the source of these problems.

As the population ages, health-care professionals are spending more time dealing with issues of mature sexuality. Doctors, nurses and therapists are aware that many patients have difficulty discussing sexual problems and might need sensitive guidance in these discussions, and therefore closely follow developments in both treatments for sexual problems.

So the first step in resolving issues of sexual health is to notice when they arise. The second step is to talk to the appropriate professional to get the right kind of medical, psychological or other therapeutic treatment to help resolve the issues. Begin by talking to the health-care professional or counsellor you trust most. If that person can't provide the professional assistance you need, he or she should be able to refer you to the appropriate source for that help.

Stay Healthy

Chapter 17, 'Finding Your New Sexuality', offers some specific ideas for exploring new sexual techniques, re-evaluating your sexual interests and maintaining a healthy, open attitude toward your sexuality. But a primary physical component of an active, healthy sexuality is a healthy vagina. Your vagina is maturing along with the rest of your body, and it's worth your while to pay some special attention to caring for this sensitive (and vital) part of your body. Don't worry – you don't need a special course in maintenance and repair to keep this part of your sexual being in order. Some very simple techniques and common-sense practices can help you maintain your vaginal health as you journey through the menopause.

First, if your sexual life involves new partners, always practise safe sex. This isn't the 1960s, and casual, unprotected sex with strangers will never again be in fashion. Don't count on your judgment or gut reaction to determine whether or not someone's infected with AIDS or other sexually transmitted diseases (STDs). Assume that they are – no matter who they are – and don't allow a sexual partner's semen, blood or other body fluids to come in contact with your vagina, anus or mouth. Your vaginal tissues are becoming thinner and easier to tear, and your immune system might be stressed by shifting hormone levels. That puts you more at risk than ever for contracting a sexually transmitted disease. Talk to your partner about his or her sexual history, use condoms and get blood tests. Safe sex practices may not seem sexy, but they're basic to survival.

Next, take steps to reduce vaginal dryness. Your vaginal secretions diminish along with your oestrogen level, which can contribute to dry, inflexible vaginal tissues and painful intercourse. Your vagina's pH balance will shift with your hormone levels, too, and that can contribute to increased irritation and bacterial infections. Oestrogen replacement is one way to combat vaginal dryness, but it's not the only method for keeping vaginal tissues moist and pliant.

fact

Sexual activity (with or without a partner) is one of the most pleasant methods for encouraging healthy, moist vaginal tissues. When you become sexually aroused, more blood flows to your vaginal tissues, stimulating the release of your vagina's natural lubricants. Frequent arousal is good for you.

A dry vagina can be lubricated easily. For additional lubrication for intercourse, use a water-soluble, starch-based lubricant, such as Sylk, KY jelly, rather than a petroleum-based product such as Vaseline, which may interfere with your natural secretions (these lubricants can be bought over-the-counter from a pharmacy). Replens and Senselle are artificial lubricants that you use two or three times a week. They coat the inside of the vagina with a non-hormonal moisturizer, which lasts for a day or two, so they do not have to be used immediately before intercourse.

Avoid vaginal deodorizers and deodorized products, scented toilet tissues and chemical-laden bath soaps and soaks. Perfumes and chemicals can further upset the pH balance in your vagina and contribute to local irritation and dryness. Make sure you drink plenty of water and eat a diet rich in fruit, whole grains and vegetables (a good idea at any time of life). Water hydrates all of your cells; drink between one and two litres every day to keep your skin, hair, bones and other body tissues fully moisturized.

Don't Forget about Birth Control

Remember, until you have gone for 12 months without a period or until your doctor has run appropriate blood tests to determine the levels of hormones your body is producing, you could ovulate and, therefore, become pregnant after sexual activity. Many women stop using birth control after they've missed four or five periods and feel that they're no longer fertile. That's a mistake; a surprise pregnancy in your mid-40s can be a tremendous problem for you and your partner. Again, be wise and use contraceptives for a year after your last period.

CHAPTER 10

Your Mind, Mood and Emotional Health

Your emotional health and physical health are closely linked. This connection is never more keenly felt than during the menopause and the years immediately preceding and following it. Many women experience a series of physical, chemical and social changes during the perimenopause that can shake their self-confidence and threaten their emotional health. But you have a remarkable ability to control the speed and severity of those changes.

Where Did It Go?

If you're nearing the age of 50 and you haven't yet begun to experience periodic memory lapses, consider yourself lucky. The busier and more stressful life becomes, the easier it is to misplace car keys, forget an associate's name, lose track of the point you were about to make and remember the title of that film starring, 'That man with the eyebrows – you know the one who married that woman who was in the soap opera for so many years... the one who's dead now... oh, it's on the tip of my tongue.' Sound familiar? As one 50-something friend once said, 'It takes three middle-aged people to tell any one story.' Multiple events challenge the memory at middle age; some of these challenges stem from the inevitable physical changes of age, and many of them are not yet fully understood by the scientific and medical communities. Although many women wonder if they're showing the first signs of Alzheimer's, the vast majority of memory loss problems are natural – and sometimes transient – responses to the effects of age, menopausal hormone changes, stress and a busy life.

Alzheimer's disease is more common in women than in men, and it strikes women at an earlier age. The symptoms, which include memory loss, diminished language and motor skills and an inability to recognize people or objects, appear gradually and worsen with age. The causes of Alzheimer's are still under investigation.

Many women report an increase in forgetfulness, memory loss and mental clarity during the perimenopause. Because hormones tend to fluctuate dramatically during the perimenopause, oestrogen deficiency used to be the culprit most often blamed for changes in memory functions. But recent studies, such as the Seattle Midlife Women's Health Study, conducted by the University of Washington, USA, in 2000, dispute that notion. In that study, researchers found that neither the age nor the perimenopausal stage of the women studied were linked to any diminishment of the women's mental functions. In fact, the study found that younger women and women undergoing hormone therapy were more likely than midlife women to report problems with memory loss.

Many types of memory loss at midlife are attributable to other, more combattable factors, such as overwork, stress, anxiety and depression. The Seattle study found that physical health, emotional factors and stress accounted for almost half of the memory loss noted in participants. Depression and high levels of stress played a key role in short-term memory degradation. Among participants in the study, only 24 per cent of memory loss was attributed to the physical effects of ageing.

tips

Although you don't have to fear that your brain will shrink up like a walnut when you hit 50, real physical changes in it can begin at this time, and you may begin to feel their impact on your short-term memory, attention span and other thinking processes. Chapter 19, 'Keeping Your Mind Sharp', offers some simple techniques for keeping your mental edge as you move towards and through the menopause.

Most medical and scientific authorities agree that age results in subtle changes in anyone's ability to think clearly and quickly, but that doesn't link memory loss to the menopause; causes for these mental lapses are tied more closely to the brain than the ovaries. First, the human brain shrinks after 50, due to a loss of water content. That shrinkage doesn't necessarily impair memory, of course, but a loss of volume in the frontal lobes can. Some neuroscientists say that the frontal lobes can shrink as much as 30 per cent between the ages of 50 and 90. Because the frontal lobes are so important to complex thinking, losses in that area of the brain can impair your ability to reason things out, maintain attention span, multitask and use your best judgment.

And the brain's hippocampus can lose some of its capabilities with age, too. This part of the brain is responsible for creating, storing and retrieving memory, and scientists now think it can lose a portion of those abilities with age. A slowing of mental processes accounts for many of the cognitive changes that you perceive with age. In other words, the information is all there and your brain can retrieve it – that retrieval process just takes longer than it used to. Metabolic changes and a diminished number of brain signal transmitter neurons (dendrites) contribute to the slowdown.

The Menopause and Depression

Are you certain to suffer from depression as you approach menopause? No, no, no – and absolutely not! Many women report that midlife brings them a confidence, serenity and inner peace that they've never before experienced. In fact, although women are more prone to depression than men (at rates two to three times higher), women in their childbearing years – years often spent simultaneously raising children and establishing careers – are much more likely to develop depression than are women in the menopause.

Nevertheless, nearly 25 per cent of all women will suffer from a type of depression at some time during their lives. And women who have a family or personal history of depression are more at risk of suffering from depression during the perimenopause. The connection between this period of transition and depression can be both physical and emotional. But to understand that connection better, you first need to understand exactly what depression is – and how it differs from mood swings and minor bouts of the blues.

fact
Mood swings are characterized by strong and sometimes rapidly changing emotional events. Women approaching the menopause often (but not always) report anxiety and panic attacks, bouts of sadness or unexplained surges of elation. These emotional swings tend to be erratic and transient, not long-lived facts of life for perimenopausal women. (Mood swings and the perimenopause are covered in Chapter 2.)

What Is Depression?

The term 'depression' is one you hear frequently. It's not unusual for people to say they're depressed by the weather, their jobs, their haircuts, their prospects for dinner or the night's television programmes. But there's a world of difference between these passing feelings of disappointment, dissatisfaction or sadness, and an ongoing state of major depression. For all of the overwrought 'depressions' you hear about every day, true depression is a real problem faced by thousands of people in our society.

Many women in the perimenopause have minor mood problems that may include insomnia, anxiety and irritability. But when these problems become severe or long-standing, these women can develop major depression. Major depression is an illness that prevents sufferers from working, eating, sleeping, studying and enjoying a full, normal life and range of moods. Major depression typically results from changes in brain chemistry; therefore, even though it can occur only once in a lifetime, many people who suffer from major depression will experience it several times.

Another, less severe, type of depression is known as dysthymia. The symptoms of dysthymia are similar to those of major depression and may be chronic and long-term, but they aren't disabling. Finally, bipolar disorder (manic-depressive illness) is another kind of depression. People suffering from a bipolar disorder experience extreme mood shifts that swing wildly between manic highs and depressed lows.

tips

If you suffer from low self-esteem, feel overwhelmed by stress or have a persistently pessimistic attitude toward life, you might be at risk of developing depression. Scientists continue to study the causes of depression, to determine whether these types of feelings are an indicator that you're prone to depression, or whether these feelings can actually trigger the illness.

Depression makes itself known to each individual in unique ways, but some symptoms are typical of the disease. Most professionals dealing with mental health recognize a number of common symptoms of depression (although they also recognize that few people suffer all of them). Here are some of those symptoms:

· Feeling persistently sad, anxious, empty, hopeless or pessimistic
· A strong sense of impending doom, with no idea of what form this awful event might take or why it will happen

- A loss of interest in hobbies or activities you once enjoyed (including sex)
- Feeling guilty, worthless or helpless
- Losing energy and feeling fatigued and slowed down
- Suffering from insomnia, early morning waking or oversleeping
- Experiencing a dramatic change in appetite or weight
- Difficulty concentrating, remembering or making decisions
- Thoughts of suicide and death or suicide attempts
- Feeling restless and irritable
- Suffering from persistent physical symptoms (headache, pain, digestive disorders) that don't respond to treatment.

Many types of medical, psychotherapeutic and alternative treatment options can help you avoid and overcome depression. To find out about those options and how to play a role in your own battle with depression, anxiety and moodiness, see Chapter 18.

The Causes of Depression

No one cause is at the source of every case of depression, but it usually is associated with a change in the brain's structure or functions. Sometimes a vulnerability to depression is genetically inherited, but depression can be brought on by physical changes resulting from stress, injury, an accident or a severe emotional event. If an individual feels at the mercy of a disease or illness, he or she can fall into depression.

Severe illnesses such as heart attack, stroke and cancer can lead to depression, as can progressive illnesses such as Parkinson's disease. Financial problems, the death of a loved one, the loss of a job, a parent's illness, the departure of grown children and other stressful changes to a daily routine also can push people into depression. Even a change of address or an abrupt change in a close circle of friends can trigger the onset of a depression that's been building up over time. Finally, hormonal shifts, such as those women experience in pregnancy, the perimenopause and the menopause, can also contribute to depression in women.

If you consider all of these potential triggers, you easily can see how some women might suffer from depression during the perimenopause. The menopause itself doesn't cause these cases of depression, but the hormonal changes of the perimenopause can combine with other natural life events of middle age to contribute to a depressed state. Women who have suffered in the past from depression or who have experienced severe PMS seem to be especially vulnerable to depression during the perimenopause.

 As you approach the menopause, consider your risks for depression. Do you have a family history of depression? Have you suffered from severe PMS or postpartum depression earlier in your life? If you have a predisposition to this illness, don't ignore feelings of depression that arise as you near the age of the menopause. Talk to a doctor, therapist or counsellor about your concerns early; don't let depression build; it's much easier to treat earlier than later.

Insomnia and Its Role in the Menopause

Insomnia is a typical symptom of the perimenopause, and it plays an active cause-and-effect role in several other perimenopausal conditions. Night sweats and panic attacks, for example, can contribute to insomnia. Long-term insomnia can contribute to heightened anxiety and feelings of fatigue, moodiness and irritability. When women don't get enough rest, they can have difficulty with concentration, focus and memory, and their overall physical and mental health can suffer.

Insomnia is a condition characterized by an inadequate amount or poor quality of sleep occurring three or more nights a week. Good, restful sleep is essential to physical and mental well-being, so every woman approaching the menopause should understand the connection between her life phase and her sleep cycles, so she can be prepared to overcome sleep problems that might develop during this time.

Hormonal Imbalances and Sleeplessness

Remember when you were a teenager and could – if allowed – sleep past noon? For most women approaching the menopause, that capacity for endless sleep is only a distant memory. A woman's hormonal balance affects her ability to sleep throughout her adult life; many women experience sleep disturbances during menstruation and pregnancy, and in the perimenopause and menopause.

Women who experience PMS (premenstrual syndrome) often report sleeping difficulties during that same, late phase of the menstrual cycle (Days 22 to 28). The physical symptoms of PMS include bloating, headache, moodiness and cramp – all of which can contribute to sleeplessness. But women with PMS report a range of sleep problems in addition to insomnia, including hypersomnia (a condition in which you sleep too much) and daytime sleepiness. As women who have a history of PMS approach the menopause, those symptoms can become even more severe.

f@ct

Women who are healthy sleepers spend 15 to 20 per cent of their sleeping hours in deep sleep. Some research has suggested that women who have PMS may spend only 5 per cent of their sleeping hours in deep sleep all month long.

Women in the menopause report more sleep disorders than women in any other age group. Many sleep problems in the perimenopause are caused by other symptoms of diminishing hormones, including hot flushes and night sweats. Although these problems may not diminish the length of a woman's sleep cycle, they can disrupt sleep frequently enough to cause fatigue and sleepiness throughout the following day.

Many doctors recommend hormone replacement therapy (HRT) or alternative treatments to combat many of the symptoms of the perimenopause and menopause, including sleeplessness. (See Chapters 11 and 12.)

The Source of Sleep Problems

Hormonal imbalances aren't the only cause of sleep disruption for women in the perimenopause and menopause. Depression and anxiety are common contributors to sleeplessness, and these problems are factors for some perimenopausal women. Remember, these problems feed each other. The less rested you are, the more powerful your negative feelings become, and the less able you are to see your way through them.

Stress – an enemy of women at any age – can also severely inhibit your ability to enjoy deep, restful sleep. A late-night trip to the toilet, for example, may be followed by hours of sleeplessness brought on by stress-induced worry. If you wake because of pain, or have a tendency to snap awake at four AM for no good reason, and lie in bed worrying about vague concerns or relatively inconsequential issues until the alarm goes off at seven AM, stress is playing a role in your sleep disturbance. All these triggers can combine to create a powerful enemy of your good health as you approach and pass through the menopause.

fact

Rapid Eye Movement (REM) sleep is the most active sleep state – the one in which dreams occur. Scientists divide non-REM sleep (about 80 per cent of total sleep) into four stages. In each stage, brain waves grow larger and slower. After the fourth stage, the deepest period of sleep, the brain waves reverse the pattern; sleep progresses toward its lightest stage, REM sleep. Typically, the cycle takes about 90 minutes.

Chapter 18 offers you some valuable techniques for recognizing and combatting problems that can contribute to (and feed off) sleeplessness. But acknowledging that sleep disturbance is part of this overall pattern is an important first step in any treatment. The next critical step is to talk with a doctor, counsellor or other health professional about these problems and their solution.

Your sleep problems may have nothing to do with stress, anxiety or tension, but could have physical sources. One in four women over 50, for example, suffers from sleep apnoea, a sleep disorder in which the sleeper stops breathing for frequent but short periods throughout the night. Snoring and daytime sleepiness are clues that you might be suffering from sleep apnoea.

Snoring isn't just something men do. It can increase with weight gain – particularly when you gain weight around your neck. If you have a problem with daytime sleepiness and your partner complains that your snoring is becoming louder and more pronounced, see your doctor. Sleep apnoea is associated with other medical problems, including high blood pressure and cardiovascular disease, so it isn't something to ignore.

More women than men suffer pain-related sleep problems. Pain from arthritis, migraine headaches, tension, chronic fatigue syndrome and fibromyalgia have been linked to sleep disruption in women. Pain can make falling asleep and sleeping through the night more difficult, but many people fail to report (or recognize) sleeplessness as a problem. If pain is interrupting your sleep, ask your GP about your pain management options.

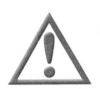

If your partner is a heavy snorer or has other risk factors for sleep apnoea, his or her symptoms could cause sleep problems for both of you. Your doctor can refer you to a sleep-study medical centre that can help diagnose the problem and recommend treatment.

Travel can wreak havoc with sleep quality and quantity, too. Many menopausal and perimenopausal women are of an age to be in professional positions that require them to travel frequently. Hopping from time zone to time zone, spending long hours in airports and on planes, rushed meetings and sleeping in one hotel after another can seriously damage the quality and quantity of anyone's sleep. If you're already having to deal with fluctuating hormones and subsequent hot flushes, night sweats and periodic anxiety attacks, this kind of disruption can make your sleep problems even more severe.

Is Your Lifestyle Keeping You Awake?

Simple lifestyle choices may be at the root of many sleep disturbances. Although you may be following the same practices you've followed for years, as your body changes in the perimenopause and menopause, you may have to become more protective of your body's natural ability to sleep. Here are some of the most common daily habits that can interfere with good, restful sleep:

- **Alcohol:** You may think a nightcap will help you sleep, but it probably won't. Drinking alcohol just before bedtime may help you fall asleep, but it's also likely to wake you up hours before you're ready to rise. Avoid alcohol for at least two to four hours before heading for bed.

- **Caffeine:** Caffeine in coffee, tea, chocolate or fizzy drinks can stimulate your brain and make it difficult for you to go to sleep and stay asleep. Limit the amount of caffeine you consume during the day, and confine that consumption to the morning or early afternoon hours. Or cut out the caffeine altogether by switching to decaf drinks or mineral water.

- **Exercising at night:** Yes, exercise is essential for good health and it's a powerful mind and body stimulant. Exercise regularly to help put your body on a natural schedule, but don't exercise in the two to three hours before bedtime.

- **Smoking:** Nicotine is a stimulant. As you've read in nearly every chapter of this book, your good health requires that you stop altogether. If you continue to smoke, however, stop at least two to three hours before bedtime.

- **Your sleep environment:** If your partner snores; if your cat or dog walks all over you through the night; if your room is too hot, too cold, too noisy or too bright, you won't sleep well and that means you'll be less healthy. Keep the bedroom temperature between 19 and 22° C (65 and 70°F). Use light-blocking blinds or wear a sleep mask. Close the doors and windows to block out sound; play calm, soothing music with the device set to shut off automatically. And finally, consider sleeping apart from disruptive sleep partners of any species (a difficult step, but perhaps essential).

Now may be the time to establish a sleep routine. Your body likes schedules, and if you can train it to sleep and wake up at the same time every day, you may enjoy deeper, more restful sleep. And don't linger in bed when you've had enough sleep: get up at the same time every day.

Putting Sleep Disorders to Rest

You can't control your body's evolution, and you probably aren't willing to tell your boss 'No travel until after the menopause', so what can you do? The most important way to promote and protect healthy sleep patterns is to pay attention to sleep problems when they arise and then take action to resolve them. If the lifestyle changes suggested in the preceding section don't alleviate your sleep problems, seek professional help to resolve them. Although surveys report that many people describe sleep problems as common experiences, many of those same people will say that they don't suffer from sleep disorders. You may think that missing an hour or two of sleep now and then isn't a problem, but you're probably wrong. If you aren't getting enough sleep – and that means at least eight hours a day for most adults – your physical and emotional health will suffer.

So if you have trouble falling asleep or are waking frequently during the night, and none of the lifestyle changes you've made have helped, talk to a doctor. You have a number of options for resolving sleep problems, including changing your diet, exercise schedule, medications, hormone replacement therapy, relaxation techniques, biofeedback and psychological counselling. Although sleep disturbances may be a short episode in your passage to the menopause, you shouldn't allow them to get the upper hand – for any length of time. Insomnia, anxiety and fatigue go hand in hand, but they don't have to grab you during the perimenopause and menopause. Protect your sleep, so you can protect your health.

CHAPTER 11

Understanding
Hormones and HRT

Hormone Replacement Therapy (HRT) has been in place for over 50 years, and although it continues to be the focus of much research and scientific debate, it remains the most studied, respected and commonly used form of treatment for menopausal symptoms and long-term health implications of the menopause. However, HRT does have risks, and it may not be right for everyone.

The Role of Hormones in Your Health

Nearly every preceding chapter of this book offers some information about hormones – their role in your body and the impact of fluctuating hormone levels on your health. But as you prepare to move into the discussion of HRT, it's important that you remember a few of the more important facts about hormones. For example, although your body produces a number of hormones, three hormones play leading roles in your reproductive cycle – oestrogen, progesterone and androgens. All three of these hormones can be used in HRT, and therefore continue to play a role in your health from puberty through your mature years.

A 1997 study of women doctors in the USA showed that nearly 48 per cent of those studied used HRT. This study, reported in the *Annals of Internal Medicine*, revealed that doctors aren't just recommending HRT – many are using it themselves.

Because hormones are such an important and widely used tool for controlling menopausal symptoms, including hot flushes, night sweats, mood swings, loss of vaginal lubrication and, later, bone loss and deteriorating vision, they are the subject of constant, ongoing medical research. As a result, rarely a month passes that we don't hear of some new development in their use, or some new question regarding their safety or efficacy.

As this book goes to press, you can assume that new developments will be emerging, and new information will continue to come to light long after you read these words. In order for you to make decisions based on the best information at hand, however, you need a fundamental understanding of these basic sex hormones and how and why they're used in HRT. The sections that follow give you this basic information, which you can use as a platform for a continuing discussion with your doctor.

Oestrogen and Its Use in HRT

Oestrogen is a growth hormone that stimulates the development of adult sex organs during puberty. At puberty, oestrogen promotes development of a woman's breasts and hips with what we think of as natural fat deposits and the resulting contours. Oestrogen helps retain calcium in bones, a function that keeps bones strong and whole during childbearing years. It also regulates the balance of HDL and LDL cholesterol in the bloodstream and helps lower your body's total cholesterol level. (See 'Heart Disease and the Menopause' in Chapter 6.) Oestrogen aids other body functions, such as regulating blood glucose levels and emotional balance. Here are some other important benefits of oestrogen:

· Oestrogen helps keep skin supple and elastic through its non-stop job of replacing dead cells and maintaining proper collagen structure (the basic structural component of skin and supporting structures).
· Oestrogen promotes healthy, well-nourished vaginal tissue to help maintain flexible, moist and elastic vaginal walls.
· Oestrogen may help strengthen the brain's blood supply and therefore aid in the protection of memory and cognitive functions.
· Oestrogen helps keep all of your body's cells and muscles healthy and well-toned.

Your body doesn't stop producing oestrogen when you stop ovulating, but it produces dramatically lower levels of oestrogen as your ovarian function declines. The amount of hormones your ovaries are able to secrete gradually diminishes in your late 40s, so your body produces lower amounts of oestrogen and other hormones. In the early stages of the perimenopause, the pituitary gland in the brain produces its own hormones to try to stimulate the ovaries to produce more oestrogen, and it works – for a while. The ovaries occasionally are able to give up enough oestrogen to trigger a menstrual period. However, in this transition a woman may experience widely fluctuating levels of oestrogen for a number of years, until the ovaries shut down completely. The body continues to produce small amounts of oestrogen, but only at about 25 per cent or less of its premenopause rate – levels too small to support the hormone's age-defying functions in the body.

Oestrogen is used in HRT to:

· Diminish hot flushes
· Keep the vaginal walls supple, moist and well nourished
· Maintain or even increase bone density
· Improve blood cholesterol levels, stimulate blood circulation and keep the arteries healthy, dilated and plaque-free to help protect against heart disease
· Help alleviate urinary tract problems and diminish stress and urge incontinence
· Help protect cognitive function
· Lower the risk of age-related macular degeneration of the eye and glaucoma
· Lower the risk of rheumatoid arthritis and Parkinson's disease

Oestrogen use may aid memory and decrease susceptibility to Alzheimer's disease, though more study is needed to determine this effect. Most studies show that oestrogen users who develop Alzheimer's have a delayed onset, compared to the general population, and a lowered severity of the disease.

Oestrogen's powerful benefits have resulted in its use in HRT for more than 50 years. In the 1950s and 1960s, many doctors prescribed unopposed oestrogen replacement, meaning that the woman received oestrogen alone, without the balancing effects of the hormone progesterone, even if she had an intact uterus. But later studies revealed that oestrogen given alone could result in the development of endometrial cancer (cancer of the uterine lining), so HRT today almost always involves some combination of oestrogen, progesterone and, in some cases, androgens such as testosterone. If a woman has had a hysterectomy, she doesn't need to worry about endometrial cancer, so her HRT prescription should involve only oestrogen.

Oestrogens offer many health benefits, but these powerful hormones can have some negative effects. Oestrogen can contribute to the occurrence of blood clots in the deep veins of the legs or the lungs of women who have a history of these problems.

If you are considering HRT and don't know your family's medical history, now is the time to ask about it. If any of your immediate relatives suffers (or suffered) from blood clots not caused by a predisposing risk factor such as pregnancy, prolonged bed rest, recovery from a motor vehicle accident and so on, you need to tell your doctor. A family history of such blood clots could indicate that you, too, carry a risk for the condition; your GP will use that information to determine whether he or she can recommend HRT for treatment of your perimenopausal symptoms.

If you have your uterus, your GP won't prescribe oestrogen-only HRT treatment of menopausal symptoms. Be aware, however, that if you self-medicate with plant oestrogens (phytoestrogens) from soya foods or supplements, you may be giving your body unopposed oestrogens. Talk to your doctor about any and all supplements and vitamins you take on a regular basis.

As you progress through the perimenopause, your body's hormonal changes take place over a period of months or years, giving your system time to adjust to gradually declining hormone levels. If you go through an induced menopause, such as follows the surgical removal of the ovaries, your menopause will be immediate and, quite probably, dramatic in its physical impact. In those cases, your doctor is likely to recommend some form of oestrogen replacement to help your body through the transition.

Progesterone and Its Use in HRT

Progesterone is an important hormone, though its benefits and impact may seem less dramatic than those of oestrogen. Normally, your ovaries produce progesterone in the process of ovulation, so most women in their reproductive years who report having regular menstrual cycles would be expected to have normal progesterone levels. Progesterone has a counterbalancing, stabilizing impact on tissue growth; it helps keep the growth of your uterine lining (endometrium) in check, for example, thereby limiting the quantity of your menstrual blood flow. In your childbearing years, progesterone also promotes the development of nutrients in the uterus, breasts and fallopian tubes to prepare your body for growing an embryo and bearing a child.

Some studies have shown that women who take oestrogen and progestogen in a HRT programme have a lower incidence of endometrial (uterine) cancer than do women who take no hormones at all.

Your progesterone levels drop dramatically when you stop ovulating. Because a woman's body produces the majority of its progesterone during the second half of the ovulatory cycle, if you don't ovulate, your progesterone supply falls. Because progesterone's most important effect in your body is its oestrogen-balancing capabilities, most HRT prescriptions for women who still have a uterus include some type of progestogen, a pharmaceutically prepared form of the naturally occurring hormone progesterone.

Progestogen serves several important purposes in HRT. It helps to mediate the growth-stimulating functions of oestrogen, so it reduces the risk of endometrial cancer for women who still have their uterus. In spite of its critical importance in balancing the effects of oestrogen in HRT, however, progestogen has its drawbacks. Some women experience breast tenderness and water retention when taking progestogen with oestrogen in an HRT programme. Other women find that forms of progestogen aggravate mood swings. And many forms of progestogen can diminish the heart-healthy effects of oestrogen, which is why doctors don't include progestogen therapy in HRT if a woman has had a hysterectomy.

For these reasons, doctors monitor HRT patients carefully to determine which progestogen type and delivery technique works best for each individual. If you have a medical history of high cholesterol or high cholesterol fractions, such as LDL (the 'bad' cholesterol) or triglycerides, discuss this history with your doctor before deciding on an HRT prescription.

More than half the women who experience irregular spotting or bleeding after beginning an HRT programme that includes progestogen stop bleeding completely after six months; 80 per cent stop bleeding within a year. Continued bleeding (after one year) may indicate a problem with the lining of the uterus, rather than a reaction to HRT. (See 'Fibroids, Polyps and Other Sources of Heavy or Irregular Bleeding' in Chapter 6.)

Progestogen can be taken continuously, cyclically (12 to 14 days every month), or in a pulsed routine of three days on and three days off. Progestogens given in a cyclic fashion usually produce a predictable menstrual period; progestogens given in the same dose on a daily basis are designed to make most women amenorrhoeic, or period-free, after one year of therapy or even sooner.

Your GP can adjust your hormone prescription or use as necessary. Because the progestogen works to prevent endometrial (uterine) cancer, don't experiment with your progestogen dosage or the number of days that you take it each month, without consulting your doctor.

Androgens in HRT

Androgens are male hormones that are normally produced in small quantities by the ovaries and adrenal glands, with the greatest quantities occurring at the midpoint of a woman's cycle. Androgens contribute to bone density (though not as dramatically as oestrogens), and some studies show that they might promote a healthy libido by fostering a desire for sex.

Androgen production also drops dramatically when ovarian function decreases around the time of the perimenopause. The decrease is even more dramatic if a woman undergoes a surgical menopause. If women have severe menopausal or perimenopausal symptoms, such as intermittent hot flushes or a greatly reduced sex drive, despite a trial of traditional HRT, their doctors may recommend an HRT programme that includes androgens.

The use of androgens to combat menopausal symptoms is relatively new, unlike oestrogen, which has been used and studied since the mid-1950s. Some studies have shown that androgens in combination with oestrogen not only slow bone loss but also may help promote the growth of new bone tissue. Some experts believe androgens help alleviate other menopausal symptoms such as hot flushes and vaginal dryness.

Androgens carry some negative risks, of course; some studies suggest that androgens can have a negative effect on blood cholesterol levels, and a few patients who take androgens can experience unwanted side effects, such as the growth of excess body hair (especially on the face), acne or oiliness of the skin. In general, androgens are added to an HRT programme only if waning libido or hot flushes are not improved with standard HRT dosages.

The Facts about HRT

Perimenopausal and postmenopausal women have a variety of alternatives for protecting their health and diminishing menopausal symptoms. The most popular and proven of these is hormone replacement therapy. However, many women are reluctant to begin HRT, and many women who start HRT discontinue it within six months. HRT isn't for everyone.

Your family or personal medical history may make you a poor candidate for hormone replacement therapy. Or you may choose to use other methods for maintaining your health and alleviating menopausal symptoms. However, your choice should be based on fact – not unnecessary fears or unfounded beliefs about the safety or beneficial impact of this treatment option. This section presents those facts.

Unfortunately, much of the information available to the public about HRT is wrong or misleading – based on questionable science and unscientific studies. Some sections of the media seem dedicated to promoting only controversial or negative findings regarding health-care issues and the medical establishment, in order to fan the public's fear (and boost their own ratings). Your trained doctor is your best source of complete information and advice about HRT, how it works, and what risks and benefits it offers you.

When you're considering hormone replacement therapy, talk to your GP, ask questions and explore alternatives. And check Appendix B, 'Resources', for a list of useful, solid sources of medical information.

Who Uses HRT?

The reasons for using – or not using – HRT vary from individual to individual, but many women who aren't on HRT have yet to make a decision regarding its use. Many women are scared off hormone replacement therapy by studies into its long-term effects. Indeed, after the results of a major trial were published in 2002, a staggering 58 per cent of women stopped taking HRT. Nevertheless, millions of women around the world do take HRT.

The decision to follow an HRT programme is an important one for any woman; as soon as your ovarian function diminishes, your hormone levels plummet. Whatever technique you use to minimize postmenopausal bone loss, heart disease, muscle and other tissue degradation, memory function loss and other effects of diminished hormones, you need to begin it before those losses build. Here's what we know about the women who choose HRT and why they choose it:

·   Though findings vary, most surveys indicate that the main reason women between the ages of 50 and 55 choose to begin HRT is for the relief of hot flushes and other vasomotor symptoms. Women who begin HRT at 65 and older are more likely to be concerned with preventing or postponing the onset of osteoporosis.

· Almost 40 per cent of perimenopausal women turn to HRT for the relief of night sweats and vaginal dryness – in addition to hot flushes.

· In the USA, a 1997 survey reported in the *Journal of Women's Health* discovered that nearly 50 per cent of those who were currently using HRT had undergone a hysterectomy. In the same study, over 35 per cent of current HRT users and over 40 per cent of past users turned to HRT as a result of surgically induced menopause. Understandably, women who no longer have a uterus have little concern over irregular vaginal bleeding.

The Benefits of HRT

HRT offers women a number of sound, solid health benefits – both for the relief of symptoms and in the prevention of some serious health threats that result from the body's loss of hormones after their ovaries cease to function.

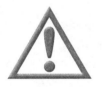

Don't overlook the importance of getting a bone density screening test! Osteopenia – early bone loss not severe enough to qualify as osteoporosis but a definite warning sign – is present in over two-thirds of the population of women. These statistics have emerged only recently, as bone density screening tests have become more common.

HRT has proven its benefit in maintaining bone health and preventing osteoporosis. Nearly 30 per cent of all women over the age of 65 have osteoporosis, and many of them don't know it until the symptoms become painfully obvious, as when a bone crumbles or snaps. Most studies show that women who use oestrogen and progestogen HRT compounds reduce their risk of hip fracture by 11 per cent for each year of HRT treatments. Here are just some of the other benefits of hormone replacement therapy:

· HRT is the most time-proven methods for mitigating hot flushes, vaginal dryness and other uncomfortable menopausal symptoms.
· Oestrogen may help to protect memory functions by improving circulation and increasing the flow of nourishing blood to the brain; early studies seem to indicate that it may help delay or prevent the onset of Alzheimer's disease.
· Oestrogen may be effective in protecting the health of the eyes, postponing or preventing the onset of macular degeneration – the leading cause of blindness in those aged 65 and over.
· Oestrogen reduces the risk of contracting colorectal cancer by as much as a third in most studies.

Macular degeneration often takes the form of a clouding of the eye's lens. Age-related macular degeneration (AMD) causes the retina to deteriorate, and it's usually noticeable first as a clouding of the central area of vision (the peripheral vision can remain intact). AMD is the leading cause of night blindness in the UK. Some doctors recommend HRT to prevent or control the onset of AMD.

The Risks of HRT

If you read the newspaper, listen to the evening news or pick up any women's magazine, you'll probably read or hear about ongoing research into the risks and benefits of HRT almost daily. Because HRT has been under study for so long, some reports about its potential risks are inevitable, but further study is needed to understand its long-term effects in full. Any medication carries certain risks. Here are the HRT risks most women must consider:

Breast cancer: A small number of recent studies suggest that long-term (more than five years) oestrogen use in HRT may result in a small but increased risk of breast cancer. Although this risk appears to be small, most doctors advise women who have a personal history of breast cancer against using HRT for at least the first five years following their diagnoses. A family history of breast cancer in an aunt on your father's side doesn't have the same impact on your health history as does an occurrence of breast cancer in your mother or sister – considered first-degree relatives. Regardless of their use of HRT or family history, all menopausal women should attend mammogram appointments when invited, conduct self-breast tests and see their doctor if they are worried at all about their breasts.

Cancer of the uterus: If you still have your uterus, you shouldn't take unopposed oestrogen (oestrogen without progesterone) for the sole purpose of relief of menopausal symptoms, because unopposed oestrogen can increase your risk of developing uterine (endometrial) cancer. HRT programmes that balance oestrogen with progestogen eliminate this risk, however, and may in fact help reduce the risk of uterine cancer even further compared to women who take no hormone supplements. If you have been treated successfully for early endometrial cancer, with a total hysterectomy, your doctor may recommend an oestrogen-only HRT regime for you after a certain disease-free interval, which is usually three to five years.

Blood clots: If you have ever developed blood clots in the deep veins of your legs or in your lungs or eyes, you may be susceptible to redeveloping them if you use HRT. High levels of oestrogen can contribute to this condition, so your doctor will want to test your current blood hormone levels and review your history to see if you are a good candidate for HRT. Low-dose oestrogen treatments may not complicate your risks for recurring blood clots, so your doctor may recommend that HRT option. Your doctor can order special blood tests that check for clotting difficulties, if your family or personal medical history raises any question about an inherited susceptibility.

Irregular bleeding or spotting is the most common side effect complaint of women on HRT, while others report breast tenderness and water retention. And, while some women say HRT contributes to migraines, others say it actually helps ameliorate migraine problems they've experienced for years.

Liver disease: If you have active liver disease or if your liver's functions have become seriously impaired through illness or injury, you aren't a good candidate for HRT. Your liver is the organ that metabolizes (breaks down) the oestrogen in your circulatory system. If your liver isn't functioning properly, your body won't be able to metabolize the oestrogen component of HRT. If your liver disease is resolved, however, the threat of this potential for an increased risk may have passed. Your doctor can advise you whether your liver function (usually based on blood tests for liver enzymes) makes you a good candidate for HRT.

The increased risk of breast cancer is slight; most studies indicate that among women who took oestrogen for five years, HRT contributed to only one additional case of breast cancer in every 1,000 women. The overall risk of breast cancer for women aged 60 to 65 who aren't taking oestrogen is low – about 350 of every 100,000 women on average. That number rises to 400 in every 100,000 for women of the same age who take oestrogen. Regular mammograms are the key to proper monitoring.

HRT may not play as beneficial a role in protecting women against heart disease as was once thought. Partial results of the Women's Health Initiative study in the USA, released in July 2002, revealed a slight increase in non-fatal heart attack, stroke and pulmonary embolus in women taking HRT, as compared to women taking placebo alone. That portion of the study is ongoing.

When the final, complete results of the long-term Women's Health Initiative are gathered in 2005, the medical and scientific communities will have a much clearer understanding of the long-term benefits and risks of HRT. Until then, discuss all your options, concerns and questions with your doctor, and make an informed decision. Don't let unspecified fears or suspicions stop you in your tracks when you're preparing a health plan for this important phase of your adult life.

HRT Options

Because HRT is such a widely used and studied method of treatment, a number of different HRT compounds and delivery methods have developed over the years. You and your doctor can determine the form that's best for you, but here are some of the most popular options:

· Pills can offer oestrogen or oestrogen/progestogen combinations that are taken continuously, cyclically or in pulse patterns of, for example, three days on then three days off.

· Patches can deliver a steady dose of oestrogen or oestrogen/ progestogen combinations every day of the month. You change patches every three to seven days, and you can wear them when swimming or showering.

· Flexible vaginal rings deliver oestrogen in steady doses to women who suffer from vaginal dryness. Some forms are available that make oestrogen replacement safe even for breast cancer patients, because the oestrogen works locally (in the vagina), and is not absorbed into the bloodstream (which could increase the potential for the recurrence of the cancer).

· Creams and gels provide topical oestrogen or progesterone doses to women who suffer from vaginal dryness. Both creams and gels are applied directly inside the vagina; some women rub vaginal progesterone gels and creams directly on the skin. Again, your doctor can advise you on the proper dose and delivery mechanism for these (and all) forms of HRT.

A new option, called low-dose HRT, has shown promising results in a number of studies in the USA, including that reported by Dr Bruce Ettinger in the August 2001 issue of *Journal of Obstetrics and Gynecology*. In that study, 138 women between the ages of 55 and 75 who had been using standard doses of HRT (.625mg of conjugated oestrogen with monthly doses of a type of progestin called MPA) were switched to 0.3mg of oestrogen daily with 14-day programmes of MPA administered every six months. The study indicated that the reduced levels of hormones were effective in reducing symptoms and caused very little vaginal bleeding – one of the primary objections many women express to traditional HRT. The protection against osteoporosis conferred by the lower dose is nearly the same as that seen with the standard dose. It is anticipated that the future trend in HRT will be towards the use of the lowest possible doses.

Designer Oestrogens (SERMs)

In the past several years, a number of artificial oestrogens have been developed to provide some of the benefits of oestrogen replacement therapy while avoiding some of the risks for women who aren't good candidates for HRT. In other words, the artificial oestrogens act like oestrogens with some of the body's tissues, but they don't act like oestrogens with others. These so-called 'designer oestrogens' are more correctly referred to as 'selective estrogen receptor modulators' or SERMs. Some doctors prescribe SERMs to combat bone loss in postmenopausal patients who can't or choose not to use HRT, but who are at risk of developing osteoporosis. Following are the most common SERMs in use today.

- Tamoxifen (Nolvadex D, Soltamox) has been in use for some years to help reduce the potential for recurrence of oestrogen-dependent breast cancer in women with a history of that disease. Ongoing study and scrutiny of Tamoxifen indicate that it isn't an 'ideal answer' for postmenopausal women. Some studies have linked it to an increased risk of endometrial polyps, blood clots and possibly pre-cancerous endometrial hyperplasia.
- Raloxifene (under the brand name Evista) has been found to maintain a certain amount of bone density, at least in some patients, without increasing the risk of breast or uterine cancer. Because it doesn't appear to have any adverse effects on the endometrium, women who still have their uterus don't need to take progestogen or progesterone

when on raloxifene. However, some studies show that raloxifene is only about half as effective as oestrogen at increasing bone density. Raloxifene's effect on cholesterol is still unknown; though it appears to reduce LDL cholesterol, it hasn't been shown to increase 'good' HDL cholesterol in the way that oestrogen does. The risk of blood clots with raloxifene seems to be similar to that of oestrogen, and raloxifene has shown no beneficial effect in reducing hot flushes – in fact it actually increases hot flushes in some patients.

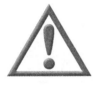

Though SERMs show great promise for the development of postmenopausal treatment without the risks of traditional hormones, none of the SERMs has been around long enough to have passed scrutiny in long-term use studies. Newer SERMs with fewer side effects are being developed.

Weighing Risks and Benefits

So how do you decide whether to use HRT, or what form of HRT is best for you? You've probably guessed the answer to this one – talk to your doctor. Reading this book and studying the other resources it mentions (see Appendix B for a list of published and online resources) is an important step toward educating yourself about the risks and benefits of HRT, but you always benefit from a professional's firsthand experience and advice when making this decision. When you see your GP, ask about the following tests and risks factors:

· Talk to your doctor about your personal and family history of osteoporosis, heart disease, breast cancer, blood clots, colon cancer and liver disease.
· Ask about a bone density test to determine the current state of your bone health. A heel or peripheral bone density test may give you all the information you need, and is cheaper and quicker to perform than some more detailed bone examinations. It is especially appropriate the first time you are screened for osteoporosis.

- Request a fasting blood test called a 'lipid profile' to find out your levels of total cholesterol, HDL, LDL and triglycerides to determine your cardiac disease risk.
- Ask your doctor about the usefulness of blood tests to determine your current blood hormone levels, or how close you are to the menopause.
- Keep your menstrual journal or menstrual symptom diary (see 'The Journey Through the Perimenopause' in Chapter 3) and take it with you to discuss the symptoms you've been having and their severity, so you know what kind of symptom relief you need most.
- Ask your doctor about alternatives to HRT and their specific benefits and drawbacks.

Part of a Healthy Menopause Plan

Hormone replacement therapy offers an enormous number of benefits for women in the perimenopause, menopause and postmenopause. But lifestyle and behaviour changes are an important part of a complete plan for a healthy life – before, during and after the onset of the menopause. No pill, patch or cream will keep you healthy if you live an unhealthy lifestyle. As you grow older, your health maintenance becomes more critical – and more demanding. So even if you adopt a full programme of HRT – or use any HRT alternative – you need to follow the guidelines listed below to maintain your good health:

- Eat a healthy diet that's high in vegetables, fruits and whole grains, and low in saturated fat and red meat. If you're interested in maintaining strong muscles, healthy bones and good heart health, your first priority must be a good diet.
- Get plenty of exercise. Weight-bearing exercise, such as walking or weightlifting, improves the health of your heart, develops muscle mass, reduces body fat and builds strong bones. The best HRT programme in the world won't protect your health if you turn into a couch potato.
- Get plenty of sleep. Sleep deprivation contributes to anxiety, depression and fatigue – the most troublesome symptoms of hormone depletion.
- Stop smoking. Smoking not only harms your health but also increases your risk for certain types of cancers that are more common in the

menopause. Smoking and oestrogen are a bad combination; do yourself and everyone who loves you a favour, and kick the habit. You can do it; QUIT is an independent UK charity whose aim is to save lives by helping smokers to stop. Visit their website at *www.quit.org.uk* or ring Quitline (0800 002200), where counsellors offer confidential help and advice, at any time during your stopping process. Alternatively, ask your GP for suggestions.

- Have regular medical check-ups. Your doctor may recommend annual checks to monitor the progress of your HRT programme. During the check-up, your GP will check your breasts for lumps; do a pelvic exam to determine the health of your uterus, cervix, vagina and ovaries; and check your blood pressure. Don't miss these appointments; they're an important part of your HRT treatment. Ask about screening for colon cancer as well.

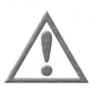

Remember to follow your HRT regime exactly as prescribed. Many people forget their schedule and miss doses. Use whatever reminder mechanism works for you – a weekly pill container, a marked calendar, notes on your mirror, or other device. If you can't find a reminder that works, ask your doctor for advice. But don't miss doses!

CHAPTER 12

Alternatives to HRT

Hormone replacement therapy isn't the answer to every woman's desire for symptom relief. Many women choose not to use traditional HRT, and others aren't suitable candidates for HRT as a result of a personal or family medical history. If you are among these women – or are simply interested in learning more about non-hormonal treatment options – this chapter provides information about HRT alternatives.

Why Some Women Choose HRT Alternatives

Chapter 11, 'Understanding Hormones and HRT', presented some reasons for choosing an alternative to HRT for combatting the symptoms and health-threatening physical changes of the menopause. Doctors may discourage women who have personal medical histories of deep vein blood clots, active liver disease and breast cancer, for example, from using HRT. If these women were to take regular doses of oestrogen and cyclic doses of progesterone, they could suffer a complication or, in rare cases, a recurrence of their prior medical condition.

Don't count on conventional wisdom to guide you in choosing HRT or an alternative. The potential for complications resulting from oestrogen and/or progesterone use differs from individual to individual, depending on dosage and personal medical history. Your doctor is the best person to advise you on this issue.

Placing Emphasis on Choice

Medical complications aren't the only factor that might send a woman in search of an alternative to HRT. Some of the reasons women cite for choosing not to use traditional hormone replacement therapies follow:

Troublesome side effects of HRT: Many women who begin HRT later discontinue its use, citing progestin-related side effects, including vaginal bleeding, breast tenderness, bloating, depression and irritability, as conditions that discouraged them from continuing the treatment. New progestogens are now available that differ dramatically from those previously available, so don't forget to discuss new pharmaceutical treatment options with your doctor.

Fear of an increased risk of cancer: Many women fear that oestrogen or other hormones included in traditional HRT treatments will increase their risk of cancer, even when they have no personal or family medical history of the disease.

Aversion to the 'medicalization' of a natural process: A 1997 survey found that nearly half of the women surveyed considered menopause a natural process that doesn't require medical management.

Do sound medical statistics support these reasons? Most studies indicate that HRT is safe and effective for most perimenopausal and menopausal women. Many women who experience side effects while on HRT find that after a period of a few months those symptoms lessen or disappear entirely. No responsible medical authority would encourage a woman with a medical history that puts her at an increased risk for developing (or redeveloping) cancer or other diseases and illness to take HRT. A calm, thorough discussion with your doctor (and possibly getting a second opinion) is the best method for assessing the potential risks and rewards of HRT for you.

The 'medicalization' question is one each woman must decide for herself. Only you can decide whether the potential benefits of HRT outweigh your resistance to replacing your body's naturally diminishing hormones. But take time to really assess your position on this issue; every time you take an aspirin to relieve a headache or use an antibiotic ointment to protect a cut or scratch, you're altering very natural processes. And if you begin a programme of taking any herb, pharmaceutical or supplement to offset the symptoms and physical changes of the menopause, you are attempting to manage the process.

Alternative therapies aren't cheap. A recent survey found that the average vitamin/mineral/nutritional menopause symptom treatment costs about £1 per tablet. If you want a good deal, seek out internet suppliers – the cost, especially if you purchase in bulk (usually three months' worth of supplies), is at least a quarter to a third less than from high-street shops.

No one right or wrong answer applies to every woman. Each individual must educate herself about all treatment options, then work closely with a trusted doctor to make this highly personal choice.

Remember, this isn't your mother's menopause. Your mother didn't have the advantages of the scientific advancements in the treatment of menopausal symptoms and the wide range of preventative medications to ward off debilitating diseases such as osteoporosis. You have a wealth of information and options available to you for managing your health through the menopause. Take advantage of the benefits of scientific advancements and research that are available for improving the quality of your life.

Although only a few studies out of thousands have shown a slightly increased risk of breast cancer following long-term use (ten or more years) of HRT, most medical authorities agree that short-term use of oestrogen/progestogen combination HRT (less than five years) does not lead to an increased risk of developing breast cancer. See Chapter 11 for more information on this topic.

Of course, there are other reasons that are a factor in discouraging women from using HRT. Some women may choose to avoid any kind of medical treatment as a result of religious or philosophical beliefs. For these women, non-medical alternatives to HRT offer the only options for maintaining physical and emotional health during the transition through the menopause.

Remembering the Medical Impact of the Menopause

When you're weighing the pros and cons of choosing HRT or an alternative, it's important to remember that you have much more to be concerned about than the physical discomforts of hot flushes or occasional forgetfulness and mood swings.

Your body's lack of oestrogen can lead to real problems such as osteoporosis and vaginal discomfort. Avoiding HRT doesn't automatically make you a natural woman or a stronger, more capable individual. If anything, it may leave you less able by exposing you to multiple health problems associated with ageing.

If you choose not to take HRT for either medical or personal reasons, you need to adopt other means of protecting your bones, brain, skin and heart as you age. As you consider alternatives to HRT, it's important that you remember the full range of symptoms and conditions you may need to combat. Some of the most common symptoms of the perimenopause and menopause are:

·   Hot flushes
·   Mood swings
·   Decreased sexual drive
·   Difficulty concentrating
·   Heart palpitations
·   Migraine headaches
·   Irregular and/or heavy periods
·   Involuntary urine release and bladder urgency
·   Insomnia
·   Panic attacks

Some of the highlighted health issues that women face as they age and their natural hormone production diminishes dramatically in the menopause are:

·   Heart disease
·   High blood pressure
·   Cholesterol imbalances
·   Osteoporosis
·   Loss of muscle mass
·   Vision problems related to macular degeneration
·   Decreased cognitive functions
·   Joint disease
·   Urinary tract disorders

- Vaginal dryness and painful intercourse
- Weight gain

Will any one treatment programme combat all these symptoms and conditions? No, it's unlikely that any single alternative treatment option will be able to solve all of the physical problems and symptoms of hormone loss and ageing. That's why any treatment option you choose must be part of a balanced, lifelong programme of healthy living and careful health management. Diet, exercise, regular medical check-ups and an active, engaged lifestyle are critical in preserving your ongoing health – through the menopause and beyond.

Don't look to any one source – especially popular consumer magazines or chat rooms on the internet – for information about the menopause. Reading this book is a good start; check the Resources section (Appendix B) for other sources of sound information.

Non-hormonal Medications

Many women use non-hormonal medications to combat the initial symptoms of the menopause, including hot flushes, insomnia, sexual dysfunction, depression, mood swings and fatigue. Medical treatments and preventatives for some physical conditions such as cholesterol imbalances, high blood pressure, bone loss and vaginal dryness are also available.

Only your doctor can determine whether you are a good candidate for any or all of these pharmaceuticals, but this section offers a brief overview of some of the most widely prescribed and effective non-hormonal medications in use for the treatment of symptoms of the menopause.

For Hot Flushes and Night Sweats

Hot flushes are the perimenopausal and menopausal symptom that many women report as the most bothersome. Hot flushes and night sweats are types of vasomotor symptoms that some women experience as their natural hormone production slows then stops in the years preceding and following the menopause. Hot flushes can be mild flushes that spread across the face and neck and pass quickly, or they can be debilitating waves of increased skin temperature that can last up to 30 minutes and leave a woman drenched in sweat and exhausted from the experience.

Night sweats can interrupt sleep or cause insomnia, and lead to fatigue, exhaustion and a diminished attention span and cognitive function. In other words, vasomotor symptoms aren't minor inconveniences for many women – they're serious conditions with both physical and emotional side effects.

Although oestrogen is considered by many doctors to be the best choice for the relief of vasomotor symptoms associated with the menopause, some other medications are available to diminish their impact. Progestogen, progesterone compounds and progesterone creams have shown some effectiveness in reducing the frequency and severity of hot flushes, as have low doses of clonidine and methyldopa, medications traditionally used in the treatment of high blood pressure. Some studies indicate that some antidepressants, for example, venlafaxine hydrochloride (marketed under the name Effexor), prescribed in very low doses, may offer some relief from vasomotor symptoms. (See Chapter 16 for information about pharmaceutical and alternative treatments.)

Many women who have a personal history of breast cancer turn to non-hormonal medications for the control of hot flushes and night sweats. Ongoing research continues to refine the medical world's knowledge of these drugs and their impact on vasomotor symptoms. Your doctor must prescribe any drugs, and is your best source of information about them.

Although each of these drug types offers both benefits and potential negative side effects, one of them may be a good treatment alternative for your menopausal hot flushes and night sweats. New medical treatments for hot flushes emerge daily.

For Blood Pressure and Cholesterol Management

Oestrogen replacement has been shown to be an effective tool for normalizing cholesterol levels in women as they pass through the menopause. Normal levels of oestrogen help to raise 'good' HDL cholesterol and lower 'bad' LDL cholesterol. Oestrogen also helps keep the arterial walls flexible, clean and wide; as your natural oestrogen diminishes, your chances of developing high blood pressure increase. Although diet and exercise are your two most effective means for controlling cholesterol levels and blood pressure, many medications are currently available to treat both conditions:

- Statins are cholesterol-controlling drugs known as HMG-CoA reductase inhibitors. Drugs in this category work by blocking an enzyme that your body uses to produce cholesterol, so they have been shown to be very effective in lowering cholesterol levels and preventing deaths due to heart disease. These drugs can interact with some other medications, and they aren't often recommended for people with active liver disease.
- Diuretics flush water and sodium from the body and can be effective in reducing blood pressure. You may have heard these drugs referred to as 'water pills', but they're much more powerful than that name would imply. Diuretics reduce the level of fluid in your bloodstream and help to remove sodium from your circulation, so they may help open up arteries and boost the capacity of your arterial system and thereby lower blood pressure against your arterial walls. However, if you do not have high blood pressure and don't have a tendency to retain water, they may not be appropriate for you.
- Beta blockers block some of the nerve impulses to the heart; as a result, the heartbeat slows and the heart's workload decreases. Doctors often prescribe beta blockers along with diuretics to control blood

pressure. Sometimes beta blockers are combined with alpha blockers – drugs that relax blood vessels – in one medication called an alpha-beta blocker. All of these medications are extremely powerful, and therefore are carefully prescribed and monitored by doctors.

ACE inhibitors are also effective in controlling high blood pressure, and they seem to work by inhibiting the formation of the hormone angiotensin II – a substance that causes blood vessels to constrict. Researchers are still trying to determine exactly how these drugs work to lower blood pressure, but some doctors are prescribing them for that purpose.

High blood pressure medications have a range of possible side effects, and most doctors recommend other methods as a first line of defence against this disease. Controlling dietary fat, salt intake and (of course) stopping smoking are the most effective weapons against high blood pressure. But for some women, medication is a necessary component of their plan for combatting hypertension.

fact

If you have access to the internet, you can turn to *www.netdoctor.co.uk* for authoritative information about most drugs prescribed today. Use the search engine to find the drug, how it works, how it's prescribed and its potential side effects and interactions.

For Managing Bone Loss

Although oestrogen is the undisputed queen of bone maintenance, medical science has made a number of strides in finding alternative drugs for slowing the bone deterioration associated with the oestrogen deficiency of the menopause.

Weight-bearing exercise and a diet rich in calcium and vitamin D are important components of any plan to maintain good bone health. (See Chapter 8 for more information.) The following medications are other options for preventing or slowing the progress of osteoporosis:

Alendronate: a biphosphonate that helps slow the breakdown of bone tissue that occurs in osteoporosis. According to the American College of Obstetrics and Gynecology, some research trials on this drug have shown that it not only helps slow bone loss but also may even build bone tissue in the spine and hip – two areas most prone to the complications of osteoporosis and possible fracture. Alendronate has been associated with irritation of the oesophagus in a small percentage of patients, but new dosages and formulations are under development that will reduce its potential for negative side effects. A new once-a-week dosage significantly reduces short-term side effects.

Risedronate: a drug that inhibits the body's ability to reabsorb bone tissue, and thereby slows bone loss. Risedronate doesn't seem to cause as much stomach or oesophageal irritation as alendronate. It also protects the bone density of the total body and reduces the risk of fracture in the spinal vertebrae and the hip, especially in high-risk women.

Calcitonin: not really a non-hormonal treatment for osteoporosis but a hormone produced by the parathyroid gland, calcitonin is available as a prescription drug. Calcitonin helps slow bone loss by slowing bone reabsorption, in a process similar to the previous two drugs in this list. Typically, calcitonin is given as a nasal spray that you take two times a day. It has been shown to be useful in reducing the risk of fractures of the spinal vertebrae in very elderly women; it does not lessen the risk of hip fracture or protect younger women.

Raloxifene: another drug that doesn't quite fit the description of a non-hormonal approach to fighting osteoporosis is raloxifene – an artificial hormone used as an alternative to oestrogen. Studies have shown that it maintains bone density in some women (though not quite as well as oestrogen) and may prevent fractures of the spine, but not the hip. Raloxifene may cause hot flushes, and although it lowers LDL cholesterol it doesn't raise HDL cholesterol. It is not considered as beneficial as oestrogen for the bone or the heart. (See Chapter 11 for more details.)

For Combatting Insomnia, Depression and Anxiety

Although thousands of people in the UK suffer from sleep disorders, insomnia becomes a true enemy of women as they approach the menopause. Hormonal fluctuations lead to night sweats and mini panic attacks that can blast a woman out of a sound sleep at three AM and keep her awake for hours. Sleep disturbances are integrally linked with depression and anxiety. Insomnia is also linked to high blood pressure, fatigue and a long list of other physical and emotional disorders.

tips

Any type of sleep-aiding medication should be used only in conjunction with lifestyle changes, including diet, exercise, a regular sleep modification routine and a managed sleep environment. Even then, nearly all authorities recommend that use of sleep aids should be short-term or intermittent.

Lifestyle changes are essential to guarding your sleep and leading a calm, rested – and energetic – life. Exercise, stress-management techniques and a diet low in caffeine and alcohol are all important components of any plan to maintain deep, restful sleep and emotional health. Although many doctors recommend HRT for the relief of insomnia, depression and anxiety, a number of medications are available to help menopausal women combat these debilitating conditions.

Hypnotics, also known as benzodiazepine agonists, have been used to treat insomnia since the 1960s. These drugs promote falling asleep and remaining asleep throughout the night. They are considered relatively risk-free, but most doctors recommend using them only for short-term treatment. Because hypnotics affect the brain's activity for a short period during the night, they can cause a loss of balance and subsequent falls in people who get up to use the toilet during the night (not uncommon during the perimenopause and menopause). The drug may also have a residual effect upon waking, making you feel tired and sluggish when you try to get up.

Antidepressants can provide true relief from the symptoms of major depression that some women report during the perimenopause and menopause. The variety and effectiveness of antidepressants have increased tremendously in the past two decades, and the development of a new generation of medications in this class, SSRIs, has broadened the applications of their use to make them more practical for many who suffer depression.

Because SSRIs, such as fluoxetine and sertraline, don't make the body produce more serotonin, but simply make better use of its existing levels, these drugs are not addictive and don't result in an artificial high of good feeling. Your doctor will work closely with you to determine whether you are a good candidate for antidepressants and which will work best for you.

If you have sleep apnoea or have to operate heavy machinery soon after waking, your doctor is unlikely to recommend hypnotics as treatment for insomnia. Hypnotics can actually make breathing even more difficult for those with sleep apnoea, and some hypnotics can continue having an impact on brain functions long enough to impair your abilities shortly after waking.

Anxiolytics, such as buspirone, are antianxiety drugs that many health-care professionals prescribe to lessen the effects of depression, anxiety and sleeplessness in many perimenopausal and menopausal women. Anxiolytics also can treat the symptoms of premenstrual dysphoric disorder (PMDD) that many perimenopausal women experience as they move closer to the menopause.

These drugs can have a slightly sedative effect, so many doctors prescribe them only for short periods of time, especially for the treatment of PMDD (when they may be prescribed for just the week or 10 to 14 days preceding the onset of menstrual flow).

Prescription medications can offer true relief from many of the symptoms and physical conditions that result from the perimenopause and menopause. But they aren't your only – and many times not even the best – answer. HRT effectively combats many of these conditions, but your lifestyle choices are always the first tool you should turn to for maintaining your health and emotional well-being at any stage of life. The following sections discuss supplemental vitamins and nutrients and a range of therapeutic programmes that can also help keep you strong, fit and healthy through the menopause.

There's a big difference between major depression and a generalized, intermittent feeling of the blues. Most doctors recommend lifestyle adjustments as the first-line defence against these and other emotional disorders. See Chapter 10 for more information.

Herbs, Plant Oestrogens and Supplements

Women have been using herbs to combat the symptoms of the menopause for centuries – in fact, only in the past century have any other options been available. As pharmaceutical science has evolved over the past hundred years, so has our understanding of the benefits of supplementing a healthy diet with vitamin and mineral compounds.

Today, nearly every woman takes some form of vitamin, herb or nutritional supplement at some time – if not throughout her life. Most health-care experts recommend that women supplement a healthy diet with certain vitamins and minerals as they approach the menopause.

As a woman's body begins changing with the approach of the menopause, its nutritional needs change. And the effects of hormonal imbalance and depletion present special problems that many women choose to address with a non-pharmaceutical solution. Many women turn to botanical compounds, plant and herb extracts and nutritional supplements to alleviate the symptoms of the perimenopause and to offset the physical changes the body can experience as a result of oestrogen depletion and the natural ageing process.

Plant substances are not inherently safer or more benign than laboratory-produced chemicals, but as yet they are not subject to official approval. Plant extracts can in fact be very powerful and can interact with prescription or non-prescription drugs to cause dangerous side effects. Don't take any substance without fully understanding its effects, and ask your doctor if it's safe for you.

Choosing Natural Alternatives Wisely

You can't walk down the aisle of any supermarket, pharmacy or health food shop without finding an ever-growing selection of herbal compounds and other botanical treatments that offer a natural approach to better health. An increasing number of botanical supplements are available for the management of menopausal symptoms. Some of these alternatives are effective – some aren't. Some of them can be downright dangerous when taken without the knowledge or advice of a trained nutritionist or doctor.

Because the sale of herbal compounds and 'nutraceuticals' – foods that also deliver some sort of medication or compound designed to offer a specific medical benefit – has become such big business, it has drawn the attention of the popular media as well as the medical community.

Frequent articles in magazines and newspapers, and on internet pages discuss the latest vitamin or herbal alternatives, and the scientific community continues to test and release results on the efficacy of these compounds for the treatment of specific physical or emotional disorders. Because botanical extracts and nutritional supplements aren't subject to Medicines Control Agency approval, each consumer is responsible for making the wisest, most informed choice when buying these products. The need for information for women seeking a natural alternative to HRT for the relief of menopausal symptoms is especially critical; the alternatives must offer relief from a range of overt symptoms while, at the same time, supplementing the body's supply of important vitamins and minerals.

Consider the following important points when you're assessing the value of choosing herbs and/or nutritional supplements for the treatment of menopausal symptoms:

Are you looking for symptom relief or health maintenance? Many herbal alternatives are effective for relieving a single symptom or for supplementing a specific nutritional need. The wider the range of relief you are seeking, the more pills, capsules, powders and teas you may need to consume. And you will need to see your doctor to assess the safety of that combination.

Have you already adopted the healthy lifestyle changes recommended for women at your stage of life? A proper diet, regular exercise and good stress-management skills are as essential for those using alternative treatments for menopausal symptoms as they are for women using HRT. No botanical compound, vitamin collection or nutritional supplement will replace these very basic necessities for maintaining your health through the menopause.

Have you talked with others who are using the treatment alternative you're considering, and have you discussed it with your health-care provider? Making a decision to use these alternatives requires that you educate yourself about all of the possible benefits and drawbacks of your choice. Again, don't think you can tinker with harmless experimentation. Your choice of botanical and nutritional supplements that are powerful enough to treat the symptoms and diminish the physical degradation of bone, muscle and brain tissue that accompanies the menopause requires your careful consideration and thorough research.

fact

No alternative medication or herb can surpass the results of modern scientific technology and the pharmaceuticals it has provided us. When deciding on a plan to maintain your long-term health during and after the menopause, get the authoritative information and advice you need to make an intelligent decision.

The range of botanical substances, nutritional supplements and nutraceuticals available for perimenopausal and menopausal women is vast. Appendix B contains a number of authoritative references for more information on this topic. The following sections list some of the most popular – and promising – herbs, plant extracts and nutritional supplements in use today for the effective management of menopausal symptoms.

What is a bioflavonoid?
Bioflavonoids are naturally occurring plant substances found in many brightly coloured fruits and vegetables, such as cherries, oranges and other citrus, grapes, leafy vegetables, red wine and some types of red clover. Researchers are studying bioflavonoids for the treatment of a number of conditions, including the control of bleeding, haemorrhoids and varicose veins.

Understanding Plant Hormones

So how can a plant or herb compound relieve the symptoms of hormone depletion and imbalance? The answer to that question lies in the chemical make-up of certain plants that contain phytohormones – natural substances found in some herbs and other plants that may help to regulate the plant's growth. Although plant and human hormones are very different substances, phytohormones (some types are referred to as phytoestrogens) can bind to the human body's oestrogen receptors; phytoestrogens may act like an oestrogen on the body or like an anti-oestrogen, depending upon their particular type and dosage.

Two of the most popular types of phytoestrogens used in menopausal supplements today are isoflavones (a class of bioflavonoids) and lignans. Isoflavones occur in soya beans, red clover and (in much lower quantities) green tea, peas, pinto beans, lentils and other legumes. Lignans occur in flaxseeds (although flaxseed oil contains only small amounts).

Natural oestrogen can be extracted from some foods, such as soya, and plant hormones from the wild yam have been extracted to create a progesterone-like cream. Some tests have shown that certain plant oestrogens offer some relief from hot flushes of the perimenopause and menopause, if the symptoms are mild. These plant derivatives are the subject of a great deal of ongoing research, as the medical community continues to test the safety and efficacy of these substances and to learn how their use compares with the effectiveness of traditional HRT in the treatment of symptoms of women with diminishing levels of hormone production.

Make sure to read some full-length texts that discuss these natural alternatives to HRT in complete detail. Use the information you gain in this chapter as a foundation for further research and discussions with your doctor.

Soya and Isoflavones

Soya is a major source of a number of important vitamins and nutrients, and it is one of the primary sources for isoflavones – a type of plant oestrogen. The North American Menopause Society has reported on a number of studies of the use of isoflavones and their role in managing menopausal health. (Some of the articles are listed in the References section of Appendix B.) Although some of the studies have been inconclusive and work continues in this area, many health and nutrition experts believe that soya has major benefits for treating some symptoms of the menopause:

· The isoflavones in soya may help reduce harmful LDL cholesterol and triglycerides while increasing beneficial HDL cholesterol levels.
· Many women find that soya reduces the occurrences and the severity of hot flashes.
· One study, conducted by Dr Michael Scheiber and associates, reported in 2001, found that women who included whole soya foods in their diet had reductions in some of the key indicators for the onset of osteoporosis.
· Some women report that an increased intake of soya isoflavones helps to alleviate their symptoms of vaginal dryness, although no long-term study has confirmed this.

With all this information and theorizing, bear in mind that the type of soya you consume has a huge impact on the amount of symptom relief you may be able to expect. For example, raw, green soya beans contain the most isoflavones – as much as 150 milligrams per 100 grams of food – whereas soya hot dogs or sausages may contain only 3 or 4 milligrams. Most medical experts recommend that if you're using soya to manage menopause symptoms, you should consume at least 100 milligrams per day (for 25 to 50 milligrams of isoflavones). In the Scheiber NAMS Fellowship study mentioned earlier, the participants ate whole soya foods containing 60 mg/d every day.

f@ct

> Asian women, who eat a diet rich in soya products, have exceptionally low rates of hip and spine fractures and endometrial (uterine) breast, and ovarian cancers. Although the Asian diet is also low in red meat and saturated animal fats, researchers are working to track down possible connections between the consumption of soya isoflavones and the low rate of hormone-related conditions.

Soya products aren't calorie-free, but they tend to be low in fat, high in dietary fibre and full of a range of important vitamins and minerals. Soya milk, tofu, tempeh and imitation meat products are just some of the readily available sources of soya. Soya sprouts, soya flour and roasted soya beans also are rich sources of soya isoflavones.

Red clover is the second richest source of isoflavones. Although some herbal teas and compounds include red clover, it's more commonly taken as a plant extract. For more information about these ingredients, see Chapter 13, 'Eating for a Healthy Menopause'.

Black Cohosh

Black cohosh is perhaps one of the most popular herbal remedies used for the management of menopausal symptoms. Native American women have used its roots for centuries for relief of a number of symptoms associated with menstruation and the menopause.

The specific means by which it works is still the subject of intense study. German women have used black cohosh for decades as a means of diminishing hot flushes, depression and other symptoms of the menopause. In some studies, black cohosh was found to lower luteinizing hormone (LH) levels by binding to certain oestrogen receptors. Double-blind tests conducted on Remifem, an over-the-counter supplement that contains black cohosh, found that some participants felt some relief from symptoms including hot flushes, depression-like symptoms and occasional sleeplessness.

More studies are needed to determine whether black cohosh is safe for women with breast cancer and other oestrogen-sensitive cancers. The side effects of black cohosh include nausea, vomiting, dizziness and at least one reported case of nocturnal seizures.

Black cohosh should not be used during pregnancy, as it may cause miscarriage or premature birth. In the menopause or perimenopause, its use is not recommended for more than six months.

Gingko Biloba

Many women turn to gingko biloba supplements, extracted from the leaf of the gingko biloba tree, as treatment for the mental fogginess that seems to descend upon them as the menopause approaches. Gingko biloba has been studied in placebo-controlled tests and shown to work better than a placebo at aiding memory and concentration. Because it improves circulation it may aid the supply of nourishment to the brain through the circulatory system.

Typical dosages of gingko are 40 to 80 milligrams (taken in capsule form) three times daily. Most sources indicate that you need to take this dosage for up to 12 weeks in order to feel the effect. Talk to your doctor for information about dosage and appropriateness for your symptoms.

Finding Out about Other Herbs and Supplements

This chapter has listed only a few herbal compounds and nutritional supplements available for the treatment of menopausal symptoms. Others include:

- Chasteberry (Latin name, *Vitus agnus castus*) is said to relieve hot flushes and vaginal dryness.

- Dong quai, believed by some to treat hot flushes, was found ineffective in recent studies and may increase the flow of menstrual blood. Other side effects include photosensitivity and photodermatitis (sun rash), and it may cause cancer or mutations or increase the effects of the drug warfarin (Marevan – a frequently prescribed blood thinner) and antiplatelet agents.
- SAMe (S-Adenosylmethionine) is said to repair damaged cartilage for better joint health.
- Ginseng root is considered by many to aid menopausal symptoms, and may have a beneficial impact on mood through its mild stimulant effect.

You'll find many other examples of herbal compounds and nutritional supplements on most supermarket, health food shop and pharmacy shelves. As recommended earlier, do your own extensive research into any supplement before you begin using it. The Resources section of Appendix B offers a variety of print and online sources for more information. And, as always, talk to your doctor for a full understanding of how these products may work for the treatment of your symptoms.

Many women claim to have found real relief from hot flushes, anxiety and other menopausal symptoms through acupressure and therapeutic massage. In acupressure, a therapist places pressure on the body at the same meridian points used in acupuncture. Many types of therapeutic massage operate on the principle that stimulating the body's circulation and lymph gland production boosts health.

Therapeutic Programmes

Women throughout the Western world are learning that many of the medical traditions from other cultures have some use for the management of menopausal symptoms. And some traditional Western therapies, such as counselling and cognitive therapy, are extremely effective for treating some of the most debilitating symptoms of the menopause, including mood swings, irritability and depression. Some of the therapeutic programmes women have found useful in treating symptoms of the perimenopause and menopause are listed below.

· Acupuncture is an ancient Chinese therapy that involves rotating fine needles until they enter the skin at specific points on the body. In a 1995 test reported by the North American Menopause Society in the journal *Menopause*, women treated with both electrically aided and traditional acupuncture showed a significant decrease in hot flushes, lasting up to three months after treatment. The US National Institute of Health Consensus Development Panel on Acupuncture issued a statement saying that acupuncture may be helpful in managing conditions such as headache, fibromyalgia, osteoarthritis and cramp – all conditions some women face in the perimenopause and menopause. This alternative treatment option is still being studied for its applications in the management of menopause symptoms.

· Breathing regulation, where women are trained to breathe deeply and slowly (sometimes called paced respiration), has also shown some promise in reducing hot flushes and aiding relaxation. For perimenopausal and menopausal women suffering from hot flushes, anxiety and panic attacks, this technique can be particularly useful. Perhaps due to the same calm, slow respiratory technique taught in practices such as yoga and meditation, some women report that those practices have also helped them in alleviating anxiety as well as the frequency and intensity of hot flushes.

· Biofeedback is a technique in which individuals are trained to monitor breathing, heart rate and blood pressure, and then change those functions through relaxation techniques or visual imagery. Studies on biofeedback have been ongoing since the 1970s, and some have indicated that biofeedback techniques can help women control hot flushes and stress incontinence.

· Cognitive therapy – a type of talk therapy – has long been used to help individuals overcome depression; many women find it an invaluable tool for coming to terms with the changing realities of their lives and health as they approach and enter the menopause. Cognitive therapy focuses on helping the individual learn to see the connection between a pattern of negative thought and depression. As you learn to replace negative thoughts with positive ones, you can break damaging thinking patterns that contribute to deepening, ongoing depression and anxiety. Many women become the victims of constant negative thinking as they approach the menopause; cognitive therapy can help break that pattern and thereby alleviate the moodiness, lethargy, irritability, sadness and insomnia that it can cause.

Lifestyle Changes for a Healthier Menopause

This chapter has saved the most important alternative for combatting menopausal symptoms for last. Lifestyle choices, including eliminating certain substances from your life; exercising regularly; eating a healthy, well-balanced diet with appropriate vitamin and mineral supplements; managing weight; and getting regular aerobic and weight-bearing exercise are essential for any woman entering the menopause, whether or not she chooses to use HRT or alternative treatments to manage symptoms.

Throughout this chapter you've been advised to seek the advice of a trusted doctor. When you sit down with that individual, the following are some of the first questions he or she will probably ask:

· 'How's your diet? Do you take any vitamins?'
· 'Do you get any regular form of exercise? What kind? How often?'
· 'Do you smoke? Do you use any non-prescription drugs or stimulants? How much alcohol do you consume?'
· 'How much stress are you under?'

So – use the following five-point plan to minimize the number and severity of your perimenopausal and menopausal symptoms, maintain optimal health through the menopause and set the stage for your healthy, active, enjoyable postmenopausal life:

Concentrate on what you can eat now, and experiment with foods you may not have tried before. Baked parsnips and sweet potatoes, for example, are tasty, rich dishes that offer good sources of fibre, vitamins and minerals. And these foods are naturally sweet, so you can throw out the chocolate eclairs.

1. **Eat a heart-healthy, well-balanced diet with the vitamin, mineral and nutrient balance recommended for a woman at your stage of life.** Feeding your body properly is the most important thing you can do to manage your menopause – and your health. Limit your salt, animal fat and simple carbohydrate intake. Eat plenty of green leafy vegetables, root vegetables and fresh and dried fruit. Make sure your diet includes ample quantities of vitamin C, vitamin D, vitamin E and calcium. Now is the time to start reading the labels on your food and eating as though your life depends on it. (See Chapter 13.)

2. **Get regular physical activity that includes both weight-bearing and aerobic exercise.** Thirty minutes a day, four or more days a week, of walking, bicycling, swimming or other exercise can keep your heart and lungs healthy, your mind alert and your spirits up. (See Chapter 14.)

3. **Manage your weight.** Obesity has become a national epidemic. According to the British Nutrition Foundation, more than 50 per cent of all Britons are overweight – and the numbers are increasing all the time. And even if you've never suffered from weight problems in the past, your body could begin to put on weight in the perimenopause.

   As you approach middle age, your metabolism slows down, so you burn fewer calories – even at rest. If you work in a sedentary job and if your idea of a good time involves a reclining couch, a remote control and a bowl of cheesy puffs, you might be feeding one of the most dangerous symptoms of the menopause – weight gain. You need to gear up for battle and commit yourself to doing all you can to maintain a healthy weight; talk to your doctor or practice nurse for advice on a diet that might work best for you.

4. **Stop smoking and don't overindulge in alcohol.** If you smoke, you need to stop now – for your health and for the health of anyone who lives with you. Death by lung cancer, heart disease or emphysema isn't pretty, quick or painless, so why increase your risks of contracting those diseases? If you need help stopping (and most people do), talk to your doctor or contact QUIT at their website at *www.quit.org.uk* or ring Quitline (0800 002200).

   And manage your alcohol consumption, too. Most medical experts now agree that moderate drinking – one or two drinks a day – can be healthy (if you aren't taking medications or fighting conditions that prohibit alcohol consumption). If you drink more than a few alcoholic drinks every day, you may be contributing to your high blood pressure. Alcohol isn't exactly calorie-free either – and the calories add up, whether you chew them or not. Moderation is the key.

5. **Manage your stress.** Stress is damaging to your health in so many ways; it can cause everything from an upset stomach to depression to heart disease. And even if it did nothing to harm your health (which it always does), stress dramatically diminishes the quality of your life. Now is the time to learn to enjoy the days and people that make up your life. Avoid the stressors you can avoid, diminish those you can't avoid, and add relaxation and rest to offset the damage of dealing with stress. Exercise, diet, ample rest and following a regular relaxation technique are your best stress busters. (See Chapter 18.)

Keeping Your Eyes on the Prize

As you approach the menopause, you may find that you gain a greater appreciation every day of your health and its precious gifts. No one can stop the ageing process – but as our bodies change, as the medical profession uncovers new treatment strategies, as science continually works to forge new understandings of our body and its processes, everything we know about the menopause evolves. As you evaluate and follow treatment options for maintaining your physical and emotional health throughout this time in your life, remember to keep an open mind and remain inquisitive.

> Remember that your goal with any menopause management plan is to maintain your physical and emotional health and to alleviate symptoms that threaten either. Don't grow complacent; the strategy you choose today may need rethinking a year on.

Follow medical developments, closely monitor your symptoms and treatment reactions and continue to work with your doctor to make sure that the plan you've chosen is the best option for you today. Nothing stays the same, and you can't afford to assume that today's treatment decision will still be the best choice throughout all your tomorrows.

CHAPTER 13
Eating for a Healthy Menopause

A healthy diet, supplemented with recommended vitamins and minerals, is your best tool for controlling or preventing some damaging and debilitating conditions that affect women during and after the menopause.

Your Nutritional Needs after 40

A woman's body goes through significant changes as it approaches the menopause; oestrogen production slows dramatically, muscle mass decreases as fat deposits increase, metabolism slows down, body tissues – including those of the heart and circulatory system – lose elasticity, and the body begins reabsorbing bone cells at a faster rate than it produces them. For many women, stiff, aching joints; mood swings; feelings of lethargy; and insomnia join the list of physiological symptoms that accompany the perimenopause. All these symptoms contribute to serious health risks stemming from two oddly disparate yet closely linked conditions – overweight and undernourishment.

The health risks of the perimenopause and menopause include an increased risk of cardiovascular disease, diabetes and osteoporosis. Add to these risks the serious health problems associated with overweight and obesity, and the challenges of maintaining your health as you approach the menopause become painfully clear. Meeting these challenges requires a diet designed to both manage weight and boost nutrition.

Does it seem as if you're eating the same amount of food you've always eaten, yet you're gaining weight? Your perception may be true; as women age, their metabolism slows down and they burn fewer calories in everything they do. So if your body is burning less energy while consuming the same amount of fuel, you will gain weight.

Many people go through life using their diets for everything but nutrition. They try one fad diet after another to lose weight; they stock up with junk food and high-fat ice cream and chocolate as 'food therapy' for overcoming anger, sadness and disappointment; they choose foods based on convenience, portability and easy cleaning. Although you may get by eating a shabby diet for a while, at some time around your early 40s you might begin to feel the negative impact of bad eating habits. And even if you've always maintained a relatively healthy diet, you still may not be giving your changing body the nutrition it needs now.

What are the nutritional needs of women during and after the menopause? Nutrition experts recommend these daily amounts of vitamins and minerals:

NUTRIENT (UNIT)	DAILY AMOUNT
Calcium	700–800mg
Magnesium	270mg
Iron	8.7mg
Zinc	7mg
Iodine	140mcg
Selenium	60mcg
Vitamin A	600mcg
Vitamin E	10mg
Vitamin D	10mcg
Vitamin K	1mcg per kilo of body weight
Vitamin C	60mg (80mg if you smoke)
Riboflavin	1.1mg
Thiamin	0.8mg
Niacin	13mg
Vitamin B_6	1.2mg
Folate	200mcg
Vitamin B_{12}	1.5mcg

Nutritional Boosts for Women over 40

Women approaching the menopause have to pay special attention to the types and quantities of nutrients they consume each day. The following list includes just some of the special nutritional concerns for women at the age of the menopause (remember that these amounts are general recommendations; women taking certain medications or combatting specific conditions may need to take more or less, depending upon their doctor's recommendations).

Free-radical damage to LDL cholesterol causes it to adhere to the walls of your arteries. The antioxidant effect of vitamin E stops the action of these free radicals, and therefore helps prevent the onset of heart disease.

- **Calcium is a woman's best friend as she approaches the age of the menopause.** Because the risk of developing osteoporosis increases as oestrogen levels decrease, women need to be particularly careful to consume the recommended amount of calcium every day. If you're postmenopausal and taking HRT, you should consume at least 700mg a day. Calcium is in milk, yogurt, cheese and other dairy products, as well as in fortified fruit juices. (See 'Eating for Strong Bones' in Chapter 8.) Nevertheless, you may need to use supplements to get the full recommended amount.

- **Vitamin D is an essential partner to the calcium in your diet.** Vitamin D helps your body absorb and use calcium, and you can get most of your recommended daily amount in 10–15 minutes of sunlight on your face, hands and arms two or three times a week. Most breakfast cereals are fortified with vitamin D. Calcium supplements are also available with added vitamin D.

- **Fibre is an important part of every woman's diet, and it's particularly important for women reaching the age of the menopause.** Women should eat 25 to 30 grams of fibre daily. Soluble fibre, found in fruit, vegetables, dried beans, barley and oats, helps keep cholesterol levels low and can help prevent heart disease and lower the risk of stroke. Insoluble fibre, the type found in complex carbohydrates such as whole grains and the skins of fruits and vegetables, provides bulk to keep your digestive system on track and help prevent colon cancer.

- **Antioxidants, including vitamins A, C, E and beta carotene, are vitamins found in a number of brightly coloured fruits and vegetables.** These are now considered important tools in warding off heart disease and some cancers, and may even reduce the deterioration of macular degeneration (age-related vision loss). Antioxidants work to stop the effects of oxidation within your body by protecting your body tissue from the effect of free radicals – molecules in your body that lack an electron, and therefore 'steal' one from other body cells. As with rustproofing treatments for your car, antioxidants block these free radicals from damaging your body's tissues. Squash, sweet potatoes, spinach, mangoes, tomatoes, red peppers, oranges, blueberries and peaches are just some of the fresh fruit and vegetable sources of antioxidants. Chocolate may also provide some antioxidant benefits, but don't forget about calories when adding it to your diet.

- **Soya and other phytoestrogens can have a beneficial effect on your body as its natural hormone production slows down.** Even though phytoestrogens are dramatically less potent than the body's natural oestrogens, they can help alleviate some hormonal symptoms, such as hot flushes. Soya protein has real benefits for your heart; eating 25mg daily can help lower LDL cholesterol by 5 to 10 per cent. You find soya protein in soya milk (7 grams in 250ml), veggieburger mix (11 grams in 100g) and tofu (10 grams in 120g), among other foods.

- **Omega-3 fatty acids are found in oily fish (such as salmon and mackerel), nuts, flaxseed, tofu and soya bean oils.** These essential fatty acids help nourish the hair, nails and skin, but that isn't their only role in preserving health during the menopause. New studies have shown that omega-3 fatty acids offer a number of benefits for cardiovascular health. Research has indicated that increasing the consumption of omega-3 fatty acids can benefit people who have pre-existing cardiovascular disease as well as those with healthy hearts and circulatory systems – especially when those fatty acids are consumed as part of a balanced diet. Try to eat two 100g servings of salmon, fresh tuna, mackerel, herring or other oily fish every week.

Eating at least one serving (100g cooked weight) of oily fish every week can reduce the risk of heart disease. Many deaths due to heart disease are the result of arrhythmias, and omega-3 fatty acids may help reduce their occurrence. One study showed a 44 per cent reduction in death due to heart attack among oily fish-eating participants.

Get It from Your Plate, Not a Pill

The best nutrition comes from food – not supplements. Although even a well-balanced diet might require the added benefit of vitamin and mineral supplements, those supplements should be used only to top up the nutrients supplied by food. If you aren't sure whether or not your current diet is giving you all of the nutrients you need, talk to your doctor. Then he or she can help you decide what (if any) supplements you need. A multivitamin mineral supplement is recommended, however, for anyone who is dieting, under stress, recovering from a recent illness, suffering from a chronic condition or trying to boost his or her immune system.

Don't forget the importance of drinking at least two to three litres of water every day. Water is essential for cooling your body, transmitting nutrients throughout your system and hydrating all your body's tissues. When you're dieting and/or exercising, you must be especially careful to drink ample amounts of water throughout the day.

Eating for Weight Management

Some changes that accompany age are linked to hormonal loss, while others appear to be linked to other natural processes of ageing. Although medical science continues to study the causes and effects of the changes women experience in middle age, some facts remain clear and indisputable:

- As women age, they tend to lose muscle tissue and gain fat tissue.
- As women age, their metabolism slows down.
- As women age, their body fat is redistributed to their abdomen and midsection, unless they take oestrogen replacement therapy, which helps maintain the traditional female fat distribution; in other words, keeping you looking pear-shaped instead of apple-shaped.

These facts aren't a signal that women are doomed to become fat and dumpy-looking in middle age. However, as you consider how to construct a healthy diet for your midlife transition, you need to keep these realities in mind.

The Facts about Midlife Weight Gain

As your metabolism slows, you burn fewer calories; as your percentage of muscle tissue decreases and fat tissue increases, your body consumes fewer calories. These facts together mean that, all other things remaining equal, if you continue to consume the same number of calories through the perimenopause and menopause that you consumed when you were premenopausal, you can expect to gain weight.

In one study conducted by the University of Pittsburgh in the USA, women gained an average of 2kg (about 4.4lb) over three years of their menopausal transition. By eight years after the menopause, the women gained an average of 5.5kg (a little over 12lb).

Although all women won't gain this much weight during the menopause, many will – and some will gain even more. Without question, exercise is a must for controlling midlife weight gain. (See Chapter 14.) But eating a healthy, well-balanced diet is your other weapon to fight off this potentially deadly problem.

fact To calculate how many calories you burn every day, multiply your weight in pounds (0.45kg) by 15 (if you're moderately active) or 13 (if you get little exercise). The answer represents the approximate number of calories you burn during an average day.

Don't misunderstand the message here; a slight weight gain at midlife isn't necessarily a health risk. Women's bodies change during their transition, and the addition of a little weight is an expected part of that change. But overweight and obesity – as determined by a Body Mass Index (BMI) of 25 or higher – are conditions associated with all sorts of health risks for men and women alike, including high cholesterol and high blood pressure. The heavier you are, the harder you must work to move, and the less you feel like exercising. Being overweight can make you feel lethargic, depressed and powerless – feelings no woman needs during her transition through the menopause. There is some truth to the ironic observation: 'The more you exercise, the more you feel like exercising; the less you exercise, the less you feel like exercising.'

In addition, the redistribution of body fat to your abdomen and midsection has dangerous implications. A large amount of abdominal fat is considered a high-risk factor for the development of diabetes and coronary heart disease.

Although slowing hormone production contributes to all of these (and many other) facts of life for most women over the age of 40, just beginning HRT treatment without making any other adjustments is not going to solve all your problems. Make lifestyle changes – a healthy diet and ample exercise – part of any health management plan.

Temporary or Fad Diet Plans Aren't the Answer

Remember, when you read the word 'diet' in this book, don't think about 'the incredible all banana and cabbage weight-loss miracle' you read about on the internet. Adopting and maintaining a healthy diet does not mean starving yourself or combining certain foods to magically block fat from being absorbed into your system. Long-term weight loss requires that you change your eating habits for good – not just until you drop that extra few kilos.

A healthy diet for long-term weight loss involves common sense: lowering your fat intake, lowering your simple sugar intake and decreasing your portion size. In general, you must eliminate 3,500 calories from your system in order to lose 0.5kg of body fat. By lowering your calorie intake and increasing the number of calories you burn through a regular exercise programme, you will lose weight. Stick to this routine as a lifestyle change, and you will maintain a healthy weight.

When you find yourself turning to food for the wrong reasons – to alleviate loneliness, boredom, fatigue and so on – stop and think of something that will really help. Call a friend, take a short walk around the block, pick up a book, go to a film, try to solve a crossword puzzle, work in the garden or write in a journal. Food won't solve any problem other than physical (not emotional or spiritual) hunger.

Good Eating Habits Aid Weight Control

A key component of managing weight gain during the menopause is to develop good eating habits. Again, it really doesn't matter what's always worked for you before; your body is changing, and your eating patterns have to change, too, if you want to avoid excess weight gain. The following suggestions may help you:

- **Avoid fast food.** No matter how easy it is to grab a meal from the takeaway or have it brought to your door by a delivery person, fast food is packed with all of the things you don't need to eat, such as saturated fats, sugar, cholesterol and salt. For the whopping 1,000 calories you may consume with that double bacon cheeseburger, you're getting precious little nourishment. Plan menus, shop for fresh produce and learn to pack your lunch (with daytime snacks). If you have time at the weekend to prepare and wrap fruit and vegetable salads, you can enjoy them through the week.
- **Try to enjoy your meals.** Sit down at a table whenever possible, and put your food on a plate rather than eating it out of your hand. Do not eat standing over the kitchen sink, and do not walk down the street eating a bacon sandwich. Take your time; look at the food you're eating, smell it and pay attention to each bite. Then you're more likely to know when you're full. Shovelling food down while you stare at the television, drive to work or read the paper by the kitchen sink is a sure ticket to overeating. If you really love to eat, do it with purpose.
- **Don't wait until you're starving to eat.** Try to eat small meals spaced out throughout the day. Eat a light breakfast, have a piece of fruit or a cup of yogurt mid-morning, eat a healthy lunch, have

a mid-afternoon snack, then enjoy a light dinner. The hungrier you are when you eat, the more likely you are to wolf down more food than you need. And the less cause you give your fat cells to get ready to stash it away. However, if you aren't hungry, don't eat. One of the biggest diet myths is that one absolutely has to have at least three meals a day. If you are not normally hungry in the morning, do not force yourself to eat breakfast.

- **Avoid eating late at night or right before going to bed.** Many people in the UK eat very little during the day, then pack it away from the time they reach home until they go to bed at night – a very bad eating habit. You're active and often at work during the day, so that's when you need your fuel. By the time you go to bed, your body should be ready to rest – not attempting to digest several kilos of recently consumed food.

- **Don't try to become a 'food reformist' overnight.** If you need a dramatic diet makeover, take it in small steps. Give up one or two of your worst food habits at a time, and introduce healthy substitutes slowly. Start small – buy sliced wholemeal bread instead of white, try a new vegetable soup recipe, set a weekly salad night, or skip the biscuits and have a handful of grapes. If you don't want to completely turn your back on your favourite junk food, try limiting your quantities – maybe even set up a timeline, with a planned withdrawal period. Don't punish yourself about your eating habits – just work to make them better.

- **Keep a food journal for two weeks, where you write down everything you eat – including quantities!** It's essential that you know approximately how much you're eating. Many people think, 'Oh, well, I had a spoonful of mashed potatoes, but that doesn't count.' The fact is that everything you eat counts, and your spoonful might be 50g, 100g or more. That crisp green salad takes on some hefty calories when you ladle on the dressing; get out the tablespoon and measure how much you use (and check the label for the calorie count). Weigh it, measure it, write it down. Then you have a better idea of the amount of diet reformation you need.

- **Pay attention to portion sizes.** A protein serving should weigh about 100g and be about the same size as the palm of your hand or a pack of cards. A serving of pasta is around 3 tablespoons, not the plateful they bring you in most restaurants. One slice of bread or a bowl of flaked cereal is one serving. A serving of fruit is one medium-sized fruit or half a glass of fruit juice; vegetable serving sizes are 2 to 3 tablespoons of raw or cooked vegetables.

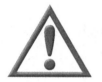

If you aren't accustomed to eating raw fruit and vegetables, add them gradually to your diet. These foods are essential to maintaining good health, but your system has to have time to adjust to digesting them. If you suddenly load your system up with an unusually high level of raw fruit and vegetables, you can have stomach pains, wind and other gastrointestinal complaints.

Sane, Simple Guidelines for Healthy Eating

Putting together a healthy diet doesn't mean that you have to have a PhD in nutrition, a live-in cook or a personal shopper. It just requires a little bit of education and a commitment to spend a little more time buying and preparing the right foods. This book isn't going to outline a week's worth of healthy meals; plenty of books do that already, and anyway, the choices are much too varied to be presented here. But here's what your food choices should represent, every single day:

· Six or more servings of whole grains
· Five or six servings of a variety of fresh fruit and vegetables
· Two or three servings of protein foods such as fish, lean animal foods, beans, nuts and seeds

With those very general guidelines, incorporate these dos and don'ts:

· **Limit your intake of fats; total fat intake should be under 30 per cent of all of your calories.** Avoid trans-fatty acids and saturated fats. Fats in nuts, oily fish, olive oil, flaxseed oil and grapeseed oil are healthier for you than are those in animal fats, margarine and hydrogenated vegetable oils.

- **Eat a wide variety of fruit and vegetables, of a variety of deep, rich colours.** Green leafy vegetables, oranges, tomatoes, peppers, squash and blueberries are some of the low-fat, high-antioxidant foods you should include in your diet. Most produce sections in supermarkets carry a wide variety of vegetables and fruit, so why stick with the same old stuff you grew up eating? Try new things, experiment and focus on nutrition.
- **Limit your intake of salt; high sodium levels contribute to high blood pressure, and too much salt actually inhibits the natural flavour of the food you eat.** If your usual routine includes salting your food before you taste it, work on breaking it. Taste your food before you add any salt. Also consider a salt substitute, particularly if you are on a sodium-restricted diet.
- **Try to add menopause-benefitting foods into your diet.** Remember the benefits of oily fish – salmon, mackerel, fresh tuna and so on – and eat some twice a week. Add soya to your diet, whether through soya milk, tofu, or soya-based imitation meats. Don't dismiss these foods without trying them. They're high in nutrients and low in fat.

Frequently, menopausal women feel that they're being forced to give up the foods they love as some sort of punishment for their age and sex. Your diet is one of the things you have complete control over, so be proud of your decision to eat the foods that will keep your body strong and healthy.

- **Be sensible about caffeine and alcohol consumption.** Caffeine has been shown to leach calcium from the body, and it can aggravate conditions such as elevated blood pressure, anxiety and tension. If you don't want to stop drinking caffeine altogether (your best choice), consider switching from coffee to green tea – many green teas have only small quantities of caffeine and are rich in antioxidants. Don't drink more than one or two alcoholic beverages a day. Excess alcohol leads to a number of health problems, and alcohol is loaded with calories. Although most health experts agree that wine has antioxidant qualities and can actually be good for you (especially red wine), keep your consumption of it low. You'll gain less weight, and you'll feel better.

Your Own Revolution

The food you eat plays a major role in determining your long-term health. As you approach midlife, you have an excellent opportunity to re-evaluate your food choices and adopt a diet that will help ensure a long, healthy, active life ahead. Food is a great joy and an important part of many of our favourite family rituals – you should enjoy eating. Maintaining a healthy diet doesn't require that you demonize every doughnut or treat the full English breakfast as if it were a ticking time bomb. It simply means making thoughtful choices about the foods you eat, and using food as a means to accomplish your health goals.

You'll never have a reason to regret improving your nutrition. No matter how many miraculous new medicines and treatments medical science develops for correcting the effects of disease or minimizing the changes that occur as we age, nothing will ever replace the marvellous health benefits of a well-balanced diet and regular exercise.

Chapter 14

Building Exercise into Your Menopause Plan

By the time they reach the age of the perimenopause, most women have developed some strong attitudes about exercise. Either they exercise regularly and can't imagine doing without it, or they've determined that exercise just isn't for them. Exercise combats many of the physical and emotional symptoms of the perimenopause and menopause, and – in combination with a healthy, varied, well-balanced diet – it's your best alternative for ageing slowly, gracefully and healthily.

Why You Need Exercise Now

A woman's body is primed for weight gain in midlife. Although becoming unfit is never a good idea, it can seem particularly damaging at this time in a woman's life. Near the age of the menopause, metabolism slows down and muscle tissue diminishes, while fat deposits develop around the centre of the body. Hormonal fluctuations can result in a variety of symptoms, including mood swings, feelings of lethargy, hot flushes and heightened anxiety and depression. Caught in a vicious circle of diminishing fitness, some women find themselves wanting to eat more and exercise less, just when their bodies need the opposite prescription.

Even those women who maintain the same level of physical activity and food intake through menopause can expect to gain weight and lose muscle tone. This decline in fitness makes even a long-practised exercise programme less effective than it used to be and more difficult to adhere to. In the Healthy Women's Study conducted at the University of Pittsburgh in the USA, researchers found that by eight years after the menopause, studied women gained an average of 5kg (12lb). The strongest predictor for that weight gain was decreased physical activity.

Does all of this mean that you're destined for fatness, not fitness, as you approach the menopause? Absolutely not! These realities of midlife change simply mean that whatever your current fitness practices may be, they probably need an overhaul when you enter the perimenopause. If you've never followed an exercise programme, if you've tried and abandoned regular exercise – even if you currently are following an exercise programme that's been working for you over the past several years – you need a new fitness plan. Following are some reasons why you need exercise now.

- Your workday may be less physically demanding than at previous times in your life. At midlife, you may have become a 'desk potato' as your job has advanced to include more managerial duties and fewer tasks that require legwork. Although you may feel as though you are constantly in motion, in reality you may only be going from sitting down to standing up more often, and not actually burning any calories.

· Your stress levels may be on the rise. As your career advances, the demands it places on you can increase accordingly. Economic and social upheavals, concerns over adolescent children and/or ageing parents and the onset of your own age-related aches and pains are just some of the stress-makers you may face at midlife. Aside from its psychological toll, stress can cause chronic pain in your muscles, feed insomnia and fatigue, and trigger weight gain.

As you pass the age of 40, your risk of developing a number of life-threatening age-related diseases begins to rise. Heart disease, diabetes, high blood pressure, elevated cholesterol levels, osteoporosis and particular cancers are some of the deadly conditions that menopausal women must guard against. Physical inactivity is a prime indicator for many of them.

· After the age of 50, your joint health and physical motor abilities can begin to deteriorate. As you lose balance and coordination, you become more likely to fall – and are less likely to participate in physical activities. Knees and hips can become stiff and painful, further damaging your interest or ability in leading a healthy, active life. The less active you are, the faster (and further) these conditions develop. If your eyesight is weakening as well, sports such as tennis and golf may become less pleasurable to participate in.

· Your body shape and your body image may be changing at the menopause. As your body takes on the natural contours of middle age, you may feel that you no longer have any control of your body's condition. A lot of people say that they just feel like giving up, but throwing in the towel about your fitness now can set the stage for a continuous and unnecessary decline in health, physical capability and emotional well-being.

Exercise Can Save Your Life

A number of life-threatening diseases become greater health risks for women as they approach the age of the menopause. Here are just some of the potentially life-saving benefits of following a regular, sustained programme of exercise:

- **Exercise makes your heart healthier:** Your heart is a muscle that grows weak with continued inactivity. The walls of an inactive woman's heart grow thin and are less effective at pumping blood throughout her system. Regular, aerobic exercise builds up the heart along with other muscle tissues in the body. The walls of a physically active woman's heart grow thicker and stronger; her heart is healthier and does a better job of pumping nourishing blood throughout her circulatory system, especially in periods of physical or emotional stress.

- **Exercise helps keep cholesterol levels down and arterial flow up:** Even moderate levels of regular exercise can lower the level of harmful LDL cholesterol in a woman's bloodstream. LDL cholesterol is responsible for the fatty deposits that collect on the walls of arteries, contributing to high blood pressure, heart attack and stroke. A regular programme of aerobic exercise contributes to clean, clear arteries that allow ample supplies of fresh, oxygenated blood to feed the heart and other body tissues.

- **Exercise helps prevent diabetes:** Diabetes is on the rise in the Western world, with increases of as much as 49 per cent between 1990 and 2000 in some countries. Obesity and inactivity are recognized as the primary culprits in the proliferation of the disease. Numerous studies show that physical activity in combination with a healthy diet can prevent or delay the onset of Type 2 diabetes, even in people who are at high risk for contracting the disease.

- **Exercise builds strong bones:** Women who participate in little or no regular physical activity can lose at least 1 per cent of their bone mass each year – even before the menopause. Participating in regular weight-bearing exercise, including walking, can slow and even reverse this bone loss.

· **Exercise can help prevent some types of cancer:** Research has shown that even moderate physical activity can lower the risk of getting breast cancer. Also, because obesity is considered a risk factor in getting endometrial cancer, exercise helps reduce the risk for that disease. Regular exercise also reduces the risks of developing colon cancer, which is an increasing threat for women aged 50 and over.

· **Exercise may help prevent or slow the development of Alzheimer's disease:** A 1998 study conducted in Cleveland, USA, found that people who exercise regularly are less likely to develop Alzheimer's disease. Physically active people who do develop the disease are more likely to develop it late in life and experience a slower progression of symptoms.

· **Exercise improves mental well-being in general:** Moderate exercise causes the brain to release more endorphins – naturally occurring substances that resemble opiates and are considered to be the neurotransmitters that make you feel good and happy. The sense of satisfaction that you get from completing an exercise routine will carry over into the rest of your day, and may help with the discipline you need to stick to your healthy diet.

Over 70,000 people suffer from hip fractures every year in the United Kingdom. Porous bones, lack of muscle strength, ailing knee joints and reduced balance and coordination all contribute to these injuries – all conditions related to physical inactivity. If you think you're too young to start worrying about these problems, think again. Many women begin suffering from impairment in walking as early as 50.

Managing Symptoms of the Menopause

A healthy heart, strong bones and a better chance for freedom from cancer, diabetes, heart disease and other debilitating and fatal illnesses are all pretty persuasive reasons to start exercising at any time of life. But menopausal women have still more to gain from following a programme of regular, sustained exercise. Physical activity has been shown to help tame many of the menopausal symptoms that women hate most, including insomnia, fatigue, anxiety and mood swings. Regular, moderate exercise has been shown to reduce stress, help alleviate the severity of panic disorders and elevate feelings of well-being. Here's a closer look at some of the menopause symptom-management benefits of exercise:

- **Exercise boosts your metabolism:** As you exercise, your metabolism speeds up, and it remains elevated for a while even after you stop exercising. The more energetic and sustained your exercise, the longer the metabolic boost lasts. An elevated metabolism helps your body burn more calories, which can help you lose weight.
- **Exercise may improve cognitive function:** A report in the US *The Journal of Aging and Physical Activity* in 2001 showed that regular exercise significantly improved the cognitive functions of individuals over the age of 50. In a research study, participants who completed 30 minutes of aerobic exercise (walking, jogging, bicycling) three times a week experienced significant improvements in cognitive functions such as memory, planning, organization and intellectual multitasking. Although researchers haven't determined exactly how exercise works to improve brain functions, they believe that the improvements may be attributed to increased blood and oxygen flow to the brain.
- **Exercise relieves depression:** In the same study that revealed the brain-boosting benefits of regular exercise, researchers also found that the relatively modest exercise programme gave participants significant relief from the symptoms of major depression. (In fact, the original goal of the study, called SMILE [Standard Medical Intervention and Long-term Exercise], was to determine how regular physical activity compared to antidepressant drug therapy in treating individuals diagnosed with major depressive disorder.) After 16 weeks, researchers found that those participants who practised the regular exercise programme had the same level of symptom relief as did those taking the antidepressant drugs. Exercise is known to trigger the body's production of endorphins – chemicals that can boost mood and alleviate tension – but researchers are still trying to determine all the ways in which exercise works to ease depression.

Body fat around the throat can contribute to snoring, a condition that exacts a toll on both the snorer and those who hear her snoring at night. Exercise can help reduce body fat, and thereby help eliminate or reduce the severity of snoring and the more serious condition of sleep apnoea – a disorder in which the sleeper experiences interruptions in air intake that result in snoring and periodic breathing cessation.

· **Exercise helps you sleep:** Many women entering the menopause are plagued by insomnia, and countless studies have shown that participating in a regular exercise programme can help you go to sleep more quickly and experience fewer sleep interruptions. (Don't exercise right before going to bed, however; exercise leaves you feeling 'pumped up' and can make it difficult to fall asleep right away.)

· **Exercise may help prevent hot flushes:** Although no study to date has shown that exercise can stop hot flushes, many studies have shown that hot flushes and other vasomotor symptoms are less common in physically active postmenopausal women than in those who get little or no physical exercise.

· **Exercise improves your endurance and makes you feel like moving:** Women approaching the menopause can experience muscle loss and joint pain that effectively discourages them from doing the things they enjoy in life – gardening, dancing and even walking in some cases. Regular exercise strengthens muscles, builds endurance and improves joint mobility and stability, enabling women to remain active and engaged in life.

Your Unique Fitness Goals

Maintaining your fitness is the most important component of your menopause management plan. Whether you intend to use HRT or an alternative therapy, whether you have special risk factors for specific diseases or no personal or genetic-based risks, whether you experience all or none of the physical and emotional symptoms of the perimenopause and menopause, fitness maintenance is your overriding priority, both now and for the remaining years of your life. If you are able to remain strong, active and well-nourished, you will experience fewer symptoms. You'll also have greater resistance to any illness or disease, and you'll progress faster and more successfully through treatments for any condition that does develop.

But what does fitness mean? There is no single universally accepted definition for the term 'fitness', because of the vast differences in individuals' genetic make-up. People inherit certain physical characteristics that affect body composition, cardiovascular actions and other important measures of good health. Heredity also plays a role in how individuals respond to exercise. But your heavy parents or grandparents have not doomed you to being physically out of shape or unresponsive to exercise. The exercise programme that's right for your next-door neighbour, or even your sister, may not be right for you. Your individual hereditary and lifestyle factors determine how your body looks and responds at its peak fitness condition.

What Kind of Exercise Do You Need?

Any complete exercise programme includes components aimed at improving three basic types of fitness: aerobic fitness, strength and flexibility. The following sections take a closer look at each of these types of fitness and some examples of specific exercises that contribute to their development.

Aerobic Fitness

Aerobic fitness involves the functioning of your heart, lungs and cardiovascular system. Aerobic exercises make your heart work harder, speeding up your heart rate and sending more richly oxygenated blood coursing through your circulatory system to feed all of the tissues of your body. Aerobic exercise has a number of benefits:

- It builds strong, healthy heart muscle.
- It increases the capacity of your lungs, so you don't get short of breath.
- It helps your body regulate cholesterol levels and keep arterial walls clean and wide.
- It builds your muscle endurance and improves muscle strength.
- It burns calories and body fat.
- It builds resistance to disease, including diabetes, cancer, high blood pressure and heart disease.

Aerobic exercises offer weight-training benefits when your body is upright and your muscles have to support its weight through the exercise movements. Aerobic exercises that include a weight-bearing component such as jogging, walking, step-training, dance aerobics, kick-boxing and skiing help build strong bones and prevent the development of osteoporosis.

Although a personal trainer can help you to determine your specific goals, aerobic exercise is effective when it raises your resting heart rate – your normal heart rate during a period of inactivity – to a target heart rate, which is approximately 60 to 75 per cent of your maximum heart rate. A treadmill or other fitness test can determine your maximum and target heart rates, but here is a general formula for finding a target heart rate:

1. Subtract your age from 220 to find an approximate maximum heart rate.
2. Multiply that number by 60 per cent; the result is your low-end target heart rate.
3. Multiply the maximum heart rate number from step 1 by 75 per cent; the result is your high-end target heart rate.

You can gauge how well your exercise has helped you achieve your target heart rate by taking your pulse immediately after exercising. Take your pulse and count the number of heartbeats per 15 seconds, then multiply that by four to get the number of beats per minute; then see how the result compares to your target heart rate numbers.

Any activity that gets your heart rate up and sustains it for 15 to 30 minutes is an aerobic exercise; this category includes brisk walking, jogging, swimming, skiing, dancing, cycling or rowing, and a host of other movement-related activities. Most health and fitness experts recommend that you get at least a moderate amount of aerobic activity every day – 45 minutes to an hour is great.

You can break the activity up into smaller chunks of time, if that works better for you. So on working days, you could spend ten minutes on an exercise bike in the morning, take a ten-minute walk after lunch, and do a 15 or 20-minute video workout at home before dinner. At the weekend, you might substitute an hour-long bike ride, a 40-minute brisk walk in a nearby park or an hour of swimming laps. If you can't do aerobic exercises every day, try to do them at least four days a week, even if it doesn't add up to 45 minutes each and every time.

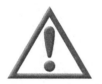

The benefits of aerobic exercise are many, but they aren't permanent. To maintain your aerobic fitness, you have to keep up your aerobic exercise – and vary the specific type, frequency and intensity of that exercise from time to time. Your body needs continued challenges to remain fit.

The choices are many, but variety is an important key when planning a successful aerobic exercise plan. Regular exercise is important, but variety within your schedule is crucial. Don't develop an everyday routine that involves the same walk, the same bike ride or the same dance routine. Changing things around from time to time continually challenges your body's muscles to meet new demands and make new improvements. Variety helps you avoid becoming bored with your exercise plan. (If you're bored with your exercise routine, you're likely to drop it.)

Some sources estimate that approximately 60 per cent of people who begin an exercise programme drop it within the first six months. Your commitment to exercise has to last a lifetime, so make it a work in progress by continually evaluating and adapting it to match your growing fitness capabilities, interests and needs.

Whatever type of aerobic exercise you choose, always precede your workout with a five-minute period of stretching and a gradual warm-up toward your full-force aerobic work. At the end of your exercise, spend another five minutes gradually cooling off with, for example, some slow walking or a series of deep-breathing exercises and long, slow stretches.

Strength Exercises

Strength training used to be considered the pastime of bodybuilders and muscle-men. Not any more: health experts today recommend weight training as an important component of the exercise programme for all people of all ages. Strength training involves performing a series of repetitive, weight-bearing motions, usually using free weights or some other means of providing resistance against the actions of your muscles. Fixed weight machines are available at most gyms and health clubs. Floor work exercises, such as push-ups and sit-ups, some yoga postures and certain Pilates mat exercises, also provide resistance training benefits for building strength.

The benefits of strength building are many. Strength training improves your muscular strength and endurance, of course, but it also helps improve the health and mobility of your joints. Strength training aids balance and coordination, and it builds strong bones – an especially important benefit for women in the perimenopause or menopause. People of any age benefit from strength training.

You have a number of options for incorporating strength-training activities into your exercise programme. Gym equipment offers a great way to ease into resistance training. These machines have adjustable weight levels, and most help you position your body properly to perform the exercises safely and get the maximum benefit from your weight-lifting action. A fitness instructor can help you construct an exercise programme that includes the use of these machines.

If you have a fever or are recovering from a severe illness, don't push yourself to maintain your regular exercise routine; gradually return to your exercise programme as you recover. It's rarely a good idea to 'work through the burn'; if any exercise feels painful or exhausting, reduce the weight you're lifting, do fewer repetitions or slow down – if pain persists, stop entirely after cooling down.

You don't need to join a gym or buy expensive equipment to get a good strength-training workout. You can buy a set of inexpensive free weights to do arm curls and lifts at home. (You can even lift tins of soup.) You can strap on arm and ankle weights while you clean the house or take a daily walk. You can create a floor-work exercise routine that incorporates traditional exercises such as sit-ups, push-ups, leg lifts and 'air cycling'. Alternatively, you can buy a home-workout video that demonstrates yoga postures, t'ai chi exercises, Pilates movements, or other types of programmes that include weight-bearing or resistance-training benefits.

In general, you perform weight-training exercises in sets of repetitions. Although a fitness instructor can help you design a programme that's right for you, most people begin weightlifting, for example, with a weight they can lift six or eight times. (Each lift is a repetition.) You may begin by performing two or three sets of six or eight repetitions, then gradually increase the number of repetitions and the amount of the weight over a period of time. In general, people who want to lose weight but gain muscle tone should do more repetitions using less heavy weights; people who want to increase strength and bulk dramatically should exercise with heavier weights but do fewer repetitions.

Most medical and fitness experts agree that strength training should make up a smaller portion of your total weekly fitness plan than your aerobic training. But in general, you may want to include at least one hour of total weight-training time in your weekly schedule. You can divide that time up into smaller segments, working 15 minutes a day four days a week, if that schedule fits your routine.

Flexibility Training

Your flexibility is determined by the length, strength and elasticity of your muscles and the range of motion of your joints. Your range of motion may be different from anyone else's – your joints are unique in their intricate make-up and conformation. But your movement patterns and lifestyle habits can determine whether you can achieve the full range of motion your joints are physically capable of, or whether you become stiff and inflexible.

Joints require movement and use in order to remain flexible and functional. Movement helps to increase the elasticity of muscles and tendons, and to stimulate the circulation of blood through the tissues of the joint to keep them well-nourished and healthy. Long periods of inactivity allow muscles and tendons to grow stiff; when that happens, your range of motion shrinks, and movements can become awkward and painful.

Flexibility is an important quality for any active life. Every time you need to stoop to pick up a child, turn around to lift something from the back seat of the car, or reach up to place groceries on the top shelf of a cupboard, you call upon your ability to stretch your muscles and flex your joints. Most sports, such as tennis, golf and squash, demand strong, flexible muscles and joints. And flexibility contributes to good balance and coordination; if you slip on a wet floor or stumble over an obstacle in the dark, your flexibility may determine your ability to recover your balance and avoid a fall. If you do fall, you'll suffer less injury and recover more quickly if your body is flexible and strong.

Obesity contributes to osteoarthritis by putting an excessive load on weight-bearing joints (such as the hip and knee). If you have this form of arthritis, however, your doctor will encourage you to exercise, both to help reduce your weight and rehabilitate damaged joints. A physiotherapist can design an exercise programme for your specific needs.

Stretching is an important exercise for increasing flexibility. Remember, you should begin and end every exercise session with at least five minutes of stretching and warm-up movements. Many exercise practices and programs, including yoga and Pilates, incorporate stretching into most of their exercise movements. Flexibility training typically focuses on shoulders, hips, knees, and the hamstrings (muscles that extend up the back of your thighs). Stretches are slow, controlled movements that gently lengthen and tone the muscles and flex the joints, to give them increased elasticity and strength.

Choosing an Exercise Programme

You have a number of options for putting together a sensible, effective exercise programme that will give you the aerobic, strengthening and flexibility training you need. It's important that the programme meets your physical and emotional needs. You need to enjoy the time you spend exercising, otherwise you're likely to lose interest in it after a short period of time. The following are some issues to consider.

- **Are you better suited to working out alone, or are you motivated by working in a group?**
- **How much assistance will you need to begin your programme?** You may prefer to begin with the on-site advice of a fitness instructor in a gym, then do more of your work on your own.
- **Can you incorporate both indoor and outdoor exercises into your routine?** Designing an exercise plan that involves as much variety as possible is one way to make sure you remain interested and engaged in it.
- **How much money are you willing to spend on gym fees and equipment?** If you sign up for an expensive exercise programme, the cost could become a reason to drop it after a short time. Look for seasonal price specials or introductory offers if price could become an issue for you.
- **Will the programme you've chosen be convenient – or even possible – given your schedule?** If you choose a gym or workout

centre that's some distance from your home and job, you'll be tempted to skip it more often. If you have to drag out heavy equipment or chase the family away from the television in order to work out, it may not take long before you decide it isn't worth it.

· **Does your programme incorporate exercises that will help you build strength, aerobic endurance and flexibility?** Don't create a programme that's going to keep you to any one type of exercise or a single routine. By varying the type, intensity and length of exercises within your programme, you'll continue to challenge your body as its capabilities improve over time.

Be open to suggestions and be creative. Play with your children. Go for a long walk after dinner. Lift phone books while you're on the phone. Put on some dance music and hop around while you fold clothes. It's all about getting off your backside and getting the blood moving again, any way you can. Every calorie you burn, every muscle you flex, every joint you move, is a point in your favour. The more you do, the faster those points add up.

Don't give up. Even if you have to step away from your usual exercise routine for a few weeks due to work or illness, get back into it as soon as time and circumstances permit. And don't let weight gain embarrass you into staying away from the gym. You're taking a positive step toward improving your physical condition, and that's something to be proud of. Changes for the positive will be gradual, so don't be disappointed if the miracle transformation doesn't happen overnight. Keep at it, and you'll see the results.

I want a programme I can work at; what's a good way to start?
Walking has the lowest dropout rate of any exercise programme. It's free, you don't need a lot of special equipment, and you can do it throughout your life. Most experts recommend walking more than three miles per hour if you're walking for weight loss. (You burn 416 calories per hour at that speed.) But don't forget to mix it up, and add other activities to build a complete exercise programme.

CHAPTER 15

Taking Care of All of You

The range of physical and emotional changes that may accompany the perimenopause and menopause puts demands on your body and mind that you've probably never experienced before. Paying extra attention to a few body care basics can help minimize the effects of ageing and keep you feeling fit and refreshed through your busy days and nights.

Appreciating the Woman in the Mirror

As you read about the menopause and the special health concerns that accompany the ageing process, you might start to feel as if your body is simply a collection of potential problems that need constant monitoring and cautious attention. It's true that the human body becomes more susceptible to certain diseases and conditions with age, and that women face special health concerns as their natural hormone supply diminishes in the menopause. But you are more than a pair of breasts, a uterus, a heart and a set of bones; you're a woman, with a life full of interests that extend well beyond disease prevention.

Every woman expects the natural changes of age to occur, but in a culture that seems to worship the physical impossibilities of eternal youth, rake-like thinness and non-stop sexual vigour and allure, maintaining an appreciation and respect for your body as it ages can be difficult. One of the benefits of maturity is a growing appreciation for the valuable things pop culture often fails to acknowledge. If you continue to evaluate your appearance and physical capabilities in comparison to those of a 20-year-old, you're destined to be dissatisfied and disappointed.

According to the National Center for Health Statistics, the average woman in the USA over the age of 20 is just under 1.62m (5ft 4in) tall and weighs 69kg (152lb). Some studies of women in the fashion industry reveal that the average fashion model is 1.8m (5ft 11in) tall and weighs 53kg (117lb). You can decide for yourself which of these is more realistic.

The most certain way to look your best is to acknowledge and appreciate the woman you are now. Then focus your attention on keeping that woman as healthy and happy as you possibly can. If you feel better, you will look better. Eat foods that are good for you, follow the exercise programme you need, keep all your NHS screening appointments, such as cervical smears and mammograms, give your skin and hair the extra care it needs, and pamper yourself with the extra rest and relaxation you deserve. Taking good care of the woman you are today is the first and most important secret to looking and feeling your best through the menopause and beyond. And part of that whole woman maintenance plan involves taking good care of your eyes, ears and teeth.

You depend upon your senses to remain in communication with the world around you, and good eyesight and hearing are essential to that dialogue. Although few women need to worry about experiencing a rapid decline in the quality of their vision or hearing as they near the age of the menopause, those functions can begin to diminish around the age of 40 or 50. Some of the physical changes of the menopause can have an impact on the health of your teeth as well. Although age-related changes are inevitable, you can minimize their impact by taking special care of your teeth, eyes and ears; by watching for signs and symptoms of potential problems; and by incorporating regular check-ups into your regular health-care routine.

tips Some medications can change your vision, either by reducing your ability to focus or by reducing your eyes' lubrication, making them dry and itchy. If you notice changes in your vision shortly after you've begun taking a new medication, contact the doctor who prescribed that medication and report the change immediately.

Monitoring Changes in Vision

At around the age of 40, many women begin to experience ocular problems, otherwise known as changes in vision. The shape of your eyeball can change as you age, and the subsequent reduction of your visual acuity can be subtle at first. A few of the most common problems you might encounter after 40 include:

- You may develop problems reading small print or seeing objects clearly that are close to your eyes. This condition is known as presbyopia, and usually is easy to correct with reading glasses or over-the-counter magnifying glasses from a chemist.

- You may begin to notice tiny specks or odd dust-like particles passing before your vision. These 'floaters' usually are just a normal condition of the ageing eye. If they become extreme in number or are accompanied by bright flashes of light, you should see an ophthalmologist immediately. A sudden increase in the numbers of floaters can be a warning of a retinal tear or other, more serious vision problem.
- You may experience problems with your eyes becoming dry and irritated after you spend some time reading or working at the computer. Again, this problem isn't unusual in over-40 eyes, and you may be able to alleviate it by using 'artificial tears' (available over the counter in most pharmacies) for better lubrication.

> If you work at a computer, don't allow your eyes to focus for long periods of time on the screen. Look up and away from your computer screen every 15 minutes or so, and don't forget to blink now and then. Overuse and strain can take a toll on eyes, and long, uninterrupted hours at the computer can contribute to the damage.

Pay attention to your vision; don't ignore developing problems. Some people experience a substantial loss in the quality of their vision before they realize that the problem even exists. That's why all women (and men, for that matter) over the age of 40 should have regular eye tests. Women over the age of 50 are at particular risk of developing eye diseases, some of which might be connected to the loss of the body's natural oestrogens. Your ophthalmologist will check for the following age-related diseases during your eye test:

- Macular degeneration attacks the centre of the retina, so central vision diminishes while peripheral vision remains unchanged. Macular degeneration can make reading and driving impossible; it's the number-one cause of blindness in women aged 65 and over. No cure for the disease is known, but its risk factors include being menopausal or postmenopausal, a family history of the disease, smoking, perhaps high blood pressure and overexposure to the sun and other ultraviolet (UV) rays. Some studies have suggested that oestrogen replacement helps postpone or prevent the onset of macular degeneration; talk to your doctor for more information.

· Glaucoma damages the optic nerve and is caused by a build-up of fluid, and thus pressure, inside the eye. When doctors can detect and treat glaucoma early, the eye can escape permanent nerve damage. Chronic glaucoma develops slowly and, in most cases, is only detectable in its early stage through an eye examination. Acute glaucoma can happen suddenly, blurring the vision and causing a number of symptoms including nausea and dizziness. Risk factors include being over 40, being Afro-Caribbean, having a family history of glaucoma, having diabetes or being shortsighted.

Doctors can't reverse the optic nerve damage caused by glaucoma, so early detection is essential. Ophthalmologists can test for glaucoma using a number of procedures. The simplest of these tests involves applying a short burst of air to your eye and determining how the surface of the eye responds to the pressure.

Your best prescription for maintaining good eye health after the age of 40 includes:

· Having regular eye tests.
· Eating a healthy diet, including your full daily nutritional requirements. (See Chapter 14.)
· Noticing and reporting to your doctor or ophthalmologist any changes in vision such as reduced night vision, clouded or blurred vision, bright flashes in your peripheral vision or changes in your perception of colours.
· Wearing good UV-resistant eye protection while outdoors – don't buy 'fashion' sunglasses if the lenses can't block UV light adequately.

Protecting Your Hearing

After the age of 50, many women experience some hearing loss, and by 65, nearly a third of all women have some decline in hearing. You might not be aware that your hearing is fading until someone you live or work with brings it to your attention. Most age-related hearing loss is gradual and can develop slowly over a period of years.

Some types of hearing loss can be the result of a physical injury, an infection, medication or the development of growths or tumours. These hearing losses are called sensorineural (caused by damage to the nerves that transmit sound from the ear to the brain), because the sensors in the inner ear lose their ability to send sound signals to the brain. Long-term exposure to loud noise causes this type of hearing loss, so if you spent the 1960s with your ears glued to the loudspeakers at rock concerts, you could experience this type of hearing loss.

Working near loud machinery, including lawnmowers and leaf blowers, can cause serious harm to your hearing. Avoid loud noise whenever you can, and when you can't avoid the noise, wear earplugs or protective headphones. You may feel like an old fogey when you move to the back of the rock concert crowd, but there's nothing young and sexy about losing your hearing.

Conductive hearing loss occurs when sounds don't reach your inner ear properly, due to problems with something other than the transmitting nerves themselves. If you have a history of ear infections, damage to your eardrum or even accumulations of earwax within your ear canal, you can experience this type of hearing loss. And as the tissue within the ear canal becomes thinner and drier, it becomes less effective at transmitting sound.

Regular hearing check-ups can reveal either type of hearing damage, but you also need to pay attention to changes in your hearing. If you notice that you're turning the television up louder these days or constantly asking people to repeat what they've just said to you, you're probably experiencing some hearing damage. Losing your hearing can make you feel isolated and out of touch with the world around you. Take steps to protect your ears and monitor changes, so you can correct developing problems before they become irreversible.

Keeping Teeth Healthy

You know about the importance of regular dental check-ups, brushing and using floss. And you also know that maintaining a healthy diet that includes a wide variety of fruit, vegetables, whole grains and necessary vitamin and mineral supplements is an essential part of maintaining full physical health, including healthy teeth and gums. But did you know that the menopause can present some special challenges to your dental health? As your body's natural oestrogen supply diminishes in the menopause, your gum tissues can become thinner and less elastic, and bone loss can contribute to the development of gingivitis and periodontitis – gum diseases in which the soft tissue of the jaw deteriorates around the roots of the teeth.

If the bone density of the jaw itself diminishes, the socket of the tooth loosens its grip and tooth loss can result. Osteoporosis in the rest of the body can be a silent process, but greater numbers of dentists are noticing loose teeth in their menopausal patients as the first clear sign of decreasing bone density in the body overall.

If you've slackened off in some of your dental maintenance measures in the past, you have to get over that tendency now. Healthy teeth and gums will help keep you feeling vital and fit and looking your best. Bad dental health habits can catch up with you as you move into your postmenopausal years. Some estimates show that over a third of all women over the age of 60 have lost most or all of their teeth. To avoid joining that group, here's a simple plan for maintaining your dental health after 40:

· See your dentist twice a year for check-ups and cleaning.
· Brush your teeth at least twice a day; use a soft toothbrush and floss afterwards. Brush for two to five minutes, morning and evening (a third cleaning after lunch would be even better) – and remember, it takes at least two minutes of brushing to remove plaque and bacteria.

- Make sure you're getting enough calcium in your diet, and limit the amount of sugar you consume.
- Pay special attention to signs of gum disease, such as bleeding or inflamed gums.
- Drink plenty of water – 1 to 2 litres every day. Water is essential for hydrating your system. It can help rinse bacteria from your gum tissue and keep the tissue moist and healthy.

Those 'water spray' tooth cleaners on the market aren't as effective as a soft-bristle toothbrush and dental floss at removing tartar and plaque build-up between teeth – the number-one cause of gingivitis. Plaque-removing mouthwashes can help soften and loosen plaque. Take the time to clean your teeth properly to avoid the pain (and potential tooth loss) of gum disease.

If you have the time to floss only once a day, do it at night, straight before you go to sleep. This is also a good time to use antiplaque or fluoride rinses; you'll have a six- to eight-hour period without eating or drinking, so your body can absorb protective fluoride and antibacterial agents.

Caring for Your Skin and Hair

If you have had no other signs of the passing years, you'll probably see some changes reflected in your hair and skin. As skin ages it loses elasticity and becomes thinner, drier and more prone to itching and sagging. Your hair becomes thinner, too; it breaks more easily and grows back more slowly. Some of these changes are due to the body's diminishing levels of oestrogen, which helps keep healthy tissues well nourished and moisturized; without it, both skin and hair lose strength and elasticity and grow thinner.

Other changes are the result of age: as you grow older, your body slows in its production of new cells and collagen production slows. Collagen is the basic bridgework, or support system, for all the fibrous tissue of your body, of which skin is only one component. Normal collagen helps keep the skin plump and resilient, providing part of the skin's support structure. Taking oestrogen helps to maintain the proper collagen content in tissues throughout your body.

The fluctuations in hormone levels you experience during the perimenopause and menopause can result in a relative increase in androgen levels as compared to oestrogen levels. As androgen levels rise, facial hairs can become thicker, darker, more numerous and more noticeable. Rogue chin hairs are a common occurrence for women aged 40 and over.

Exposure to the sun is another culprit in the deterioration of your skin's elasticity and moisture. The ultraviolet rays of the sun begin damaging the skin of young children; as sun exposure builds over the years, the damage becomes increasingly severe and apparent. Proper use of sunscreen with enough UV protection (factor 15 or higher) and using hats or caps and sunglasses to shade your face and eyes may delay or prevent this damage.

Skin Care Basics

Your diet, the amount of rest you get every day, the level of stress you're subjected to, and the types of pollutants that exist in your environment all play a role in the health and vitality of your skin. Although your skin is unique, most women need to moisturize their skin more frequently after the age of 40. A number of creams, lotions and even some prescription drugs are available today for nourishing and healing ageing skin:

· Creams and lotions containing alpha hydroxy acids (AHAs) dissolve the upper layer of skin that has suffered the most damage, revealing fresher, plumper skin beneath. These products won't eliminate deep wrinkles or age spots, but they can make the skin look and feel fresher. Some women experience skin rashes and irritations when using these creams and lotions. Women with sensitive skin or rosacea should not use these products without the advice of a GP or dermatologist.

- Oils, creams and lotions containing antioxidants and vitamin derivatives may help protect collagen, moisturize the skin's upper layer and help diminish the visible signs of fine wrinkles. Vitamins C, E and A are typical antioxidants used in these products.
- Retinol, a vitamin A derivative, is also a common anti-ageing formula component. Prescription drugs such as Retin-A are marketed to reduce fine-line wrinkles, build collagen and help fade age spots. As with other skin care products, some women report that these drugs help their skin look younger and fresher, but results vary. Talk to a dermatologist to learn more.

You also have some very basic tools at your disposal for protecting your skin. No matter what other skin care treatments you use, follow these basic practices to protect your skin and keep it looking its best:

- Drink at least 1 litre of water every day.
- Stop smoking – smoking ages the skin, breaks down its collagen structure and increases wrinkles and sagging, especially around the mouth and the eyes.
- Any time you go outdoors, use a sunscreen of factor 15 or higher, even if skies are overcast.
- Maintain a daily skin care routine of gentle washing in lukewarm water, using a very mild soap. Avoid soaps with excessive perfumes and deodorizing chemicals, and don't scrub your skin! Use a moisturizer everywhere your skin feels dry, but especially around your eyes, mouth, throat and hands.

Keeping Your Hair Healthy and Strong

The changes in your hair growth and health in the perimenopause and postmenopause can seem very unfair: the hair on your scalp starts to become thin, sparse and grey, while some of the previously fine, pale hairs on your face grow thicker and darker. You can pull out unwanted facial hair with tweezers, wax or chemically dissolve it, or use electrolysis to permanently destroy the hair follicles. (Some women experience skin irritation from electrolysis.) Although some of these changes are inevitable with age, you have a number of options available to you for preserving the health and vitality of your hair.

First, the basics: keep your hair trimmed to remove split, brittle ends and encourage volume. Some colour treatments can give the effect of fullness, and volumizing shampoos can coat thin hair to give it extra body. When you shampoo, use warm – not hot – water, and limit blow-drying as much as possible. Some deep conditioning treatments, used every few weeks, can help keep hair strong and less prone to breaking and splitting.

Your hair reflects your nutrition, too. Don't forget to include a wide variety of fresh fruit and vegetables in your diet, and take vitamin supplements to make sure that you're getting all the recommended nutrients every day. Proper hydration is essential to healthy hair, so don't forget to drink the recommended 2 litres or more of water every day.

Some prescription drugs are available to help manage menopausal hair problems:

- Minoxidil (marketed under the name Regaine) works to stimulate hair follicles that may have grown dormant. Minoxidil can help restore lost hair by 10 per cent or more, according to some estimates.
- Eflornithine may help stop unwanted hair growth. Eflornithine (marketed in its topical form as Vaniqa) can be applied as a cream directly to the area where unwanted hair growth occurs. The drug inhibits the production of an enzyme that contributes to hair growth; as a result, the drug slows the growth of unwanted hair.

Thinning, dry, brittle hair may be more than a natural sign of age. Some medications and certain systemic illnesses, such as a thyroid disorder, can also cause hair to lose its strength and vitality – even to the point of causing dramatic hair loss. If this is the case, talk to your doctor about noticeable changes to your hair's strength and appearance; don't assume you're just looking your age.

These hair and skin preparations and prescriptions take weeks, if not months, to show a result. Don't be discouraged and give up your treatment programme if you don't see results overnight.

Making Time for Rest and Relaxation

Stress and fatigue are the enemies of your health, vitality and natural beauty. Many of the most common symptoms of the perimenopause and menopause, including mood swings, hot flushes, headaches, high blood pressure and lethargy, are caused or complicated by excess stress and lack of rest. You may be accustomed to thinking of your body as a non-stop powerhouse that thrives on stress and performs best under pressure. Even if that belief was true when you were 20, it doesn't hold true now. Your body and mind need adequate amounts of rest and enjoyment, especially during the years preceding the menopause.

If you don't find positive ways to relax and reduce stress, you may easily find negative ways to do so. Many people turn to food, alcohol or drugs to help ease stress or avoid feelings of low self-esteem, anxiety or boredom. When you feel that taking time for leisure and relaxation is an indulgence, think about the potential dangers of some other indulgences you could turn to.

Participating in regular aerobic and strengthening exercise is critical for maintaining your body's ability to enjoy healthy, restful sleep. But part of your weekly fitness plan should also include some time – every day – for relaxation. Even 30 minutes of planned relaxation a day can make a big difference in your physical and mental health. Determine what relaxation technique works best for you – many activities can soothe your mind and rejuvenate feelings of well-being. Here are just a few suggestions:

· Mind/body practices, such as relaxation exercises, meditation, yoga or t'ai chi (see Chapter 14)

- Reading, listening to music or playing an instrument
- Talking with friends, spending time with your partner, playing catch with your children, walking your dog
- Soaking your feet, taking a leisurely bath or giving yourself a facial
- Gardening, painting, writing in a journal
- Reading religious texts or practising your faith

If your life is crowded, busy and packed with a long to-do list of weighty responsibilities, you may need to force yourself to sit back, relax and enjoy life for a few moments every day. But you'll do yourself and your family, job and friends a favour by keeping your body and mind well rested and relaxed. You won't look good, feel good or perform well if you starve yourself of leisure. As you move through the menopause, you have to consider rest and relaxation an essential luxury for a physically and emotionally healthy life.

 Stress can lead to insomnia and the long list of health problems associated with a lack of healthy, restful sleep. For important information on how to promote good sleep, see Chapter 10, 'Your Mind, Mood and Emotional Health'.

CHAPTER 16

Coping
with Hot Flushes

When women seek relief of menopause symptoms, hot flushes are the symptom they cite most often. Although hot flushes do fade in time, severe vasomotor symptoms can disrupt both the waking and sleeping hours of your busy life for several years. Fortunately, you have many options to choose from for reducing or eliminating hot flushes, but you need to choose these carefully and in consultation with your doctor.

A Short Review of the Hot Flush Facts

Nearly 90 per cent of all women passing through the stages of menopause will experience hot flushes during some part of the transition. Although hot flushes are a common symptom of the menopause, in many cases they are minor inconveniences rather than alarming problems. Hot flushes typically begin with an increase in heart rate and a slight feeling of warmth, usually occurring in the face, neck and shoulders. Women describe hot flushes differently, depending upon the frequency and severity of their own experience.

Mild or moderate hot flushes may last anywhere from one to 15 minutes, and cause feelings of mild warmth, accompanied by light perspiration and a slightly dry mouth. After the flush passes, the skin may feel slightly clammy. Mild hot flushes pass with little or no impact on general feelings of well-being.

Most women begin having hot flushes within the first year after they stop menstruating. Women who undergo induced or surgical menopause are most prone to suffering hot flushes. The immediate drop in hormone production that follows removal of the ovaries or a temporary interruption in their functions can result in sudden and severe vasomotor symptoms.

Severe hot flushes can last for up to 45 minutes, and cause the skin temperature to rise dramatically. The face, neck and throat can become flushed and red, and the body can break out in heavy perspiration. A woman experiencing a severe hot flush can have difficulty breathing, and the hot flush can induce panic attacks and distress. Afterwards, the woman may be left with a headache, some nausea and a general feeling of anxiety and exhaustion.

If hot flushes are severe or long-lasting, they can contribute to a number of issues that can have a negative effect on your health and well-being. Hot flushes that occur at night – often known as night sweats – can interrupt sleep and lead to daytime fatigue, exhaustion and decreased cognitive abilities. The fear of breaking into a clothes-drenching sweat during business meetings or social events can lead to anxiety and even depression.

When hot flushes degrade the quality of your sleep or prevent you from being fully functional during the day, you need to take action. Some of the most widely recommended and effective methods for easing or eliminating the frequency and severity of these symptoms are discussed later in this chapter.

What's Happening When You Have a Hot Flush?

Hot flushes are connected to changes in oestrogen levels, although the specific cause-and-effect relationship is still under study. Flagging levels of oestrogen may set the stage for hot flushes, but actual hot flushes are the result of a sudden resetting of the body's thermostat.

If your brain senses that your body is too hot – for any reason, including low oestrogen, increased blood flow to the brain, a high ambient temperature or even the ingestion of hot, spicy foods – it sends out a signal that your body needs to cool off. In response, your pituitary gland sends out luteinizing hormone (LH), which causes the blood vessels near your skin's surface to dilate to release heat through your skin. This heat-releasing action makes your skin temperature (and your body temperature) rise, followed by an increase in perspiration. The perspiration helps to cool the skin, which can result in a clammy feeling. If you've perspired heavily, you may be left damp and even chilly. Your body temperature drops and your blood vessels constrict – and if you are damp and cold, you may begin to shiver. That's the hot flush in action.

If you suffer from severe hot flushes, it's not unusual to have feelings of nausea, headache and weakness afterwards — especially when hot flushes last for 30 or 45 minutes. If your feelings of intense heat last for longer than an hour, you may not be experiencing symptoms of the perimenopause or menopause, and you should consult your doctor.

Common Hot Flush Triggers

So hot flushes are signals that your body may be suffering fluctuating levels of oestrogen or that your oestrogen levels have declined dramatically. But other factors can cause hot flushes or contribute to their severity. Many women find, for example, that they have hot flushes during periods of anxiety and nervousness; other studies have found that some prescription antihypertensive and antianxiety medications may also cause hot flushes. As mentioned earlier, hot flushes may indicate that your body is reacting to certain foods or beverages or even the temperature of the air around you – some women report their hot flushes are more severe and last longer when they occur during hot weather or in a hot room.

How Many, How Bad, How Long?

Although many women don't seem to notice hot flushes until after the menopause has occurred, many others begin having them during the perimenopause, with 48 being an average age for the onset of hot flushes.

A number of studies have been conducted on the prevalence, frequency and intensity of hot flushes in perimenopausal and menopausal women. In general, women who experience hot flushes start having them at least one year before the menopause, and continue to have them for one to six years.

The American College of Obstetricians and Gynecologists's publication *Managing Menopause* lists the findings of one study, in which 501 women were asked about the frequency and severity of their hot flushes. Of those participating in the study, 87 per cent reported having one or more flushes per day; of those experiencing multiple daily hot flushes, the numbers of incidents per day ranged from five to 50, with a third of the women reporting more than ten. Another study reported a lower frequency of hot flushes – participants had an average of only three or four flushes a day. That study also showed that, on average, hot flushes lasted about three and a half minutes, although some can come and go in no more than five seconds. And in nearly every study, almost three-quarters of the respondents said their hot flushes were mild, moderate or only variably intense.

Techniques for Turning Down the Heat

A number of treatment options to help you alleviate – or even eliminate – hot flushes caused by the onset of the menopause are discussed later in this chapter. But you have a variety of first-defence techniques available to you that don't require any special medication or therapeutic programme. Try these techniques to avoid hot flushes or minimize their severity:

- **Avoid triggering foods and drinks.** Spicy foods – foods heavy in capsaicin, the heat-inducing chemical in cayenne and other hot peppers – can contribute to hot flushes. Caffeine and alcohol are also common triggers, so you should avoid caffeinated beverages, excessive amounts of chocolate and alcoholic beverages if you are suffering from hot flushes.
- **Drink plenty of water during the day – at least 2 litres.** Keep a glass of iced water with you during meetings and conferences, and put a thermal-lined drink container of iced water on your bedside table, ready to help cool down raging hot flushes.
- **Get at least 30 minutes of exercise every day.** Regular exercise is an integral part of any healthy lifestyle, but it can offer specific relief from vasomotor symptoms. Exercise, including stretching, aerobic and weight-bearing activities, has been shown to cut down on the frequency of hot flushes, and may even help limit the length and severity of hot flushes that occur. Regular exercise also promotes a general feeling of well-being that can help reduce anxiety and stress that can contribute to hot flushes.
- **Wear layers of moisture-absorbing clothing.** When a hot flush strikes, take off one or more layers of clothing to help cool your skin temperature quickly. Cotton fabrics are particularly helpful in allowing adequate air to reach the skin, and they're good at absorbing perspiration. Cotton wicks moisture away from the skin and into the air, so both you and your clothing can dry more quickly. Tightly woven synthetic fabrics can hold in both body heat and moisture, making the hot flush more severe and its effects longer lasting.
- **Keep your thermostat turned down – 21°C (70°F) or lower during the day, and 18°C (65°F) or lower at night.** Lower temperatures can help ward off the onset of hot flushes, and you'll cool off more quickly

from those that do occur when the air around you is cool. Keep an electric or battery-operated fan handy, and turn it on whenever necessary. If you suffer from night sweats, it's especially important that you keep your bedroom temperature cool; in summer use a fan to keep the air moving around your room.

- **Manage stress to the best of your ability.** Avoid stress if you can, but be prepared for stressful situations you can't sidestep. Deep breathing exercises, meditation, yoga and visualization are all helpful techniques for boosting your ability to remain calm and centred throughout your day. Massage therapy and acupressure can also help you manage your response to stress and reduce the frequency of stress-induced hot flushes.

If a hot flush strikes, you may get some quick relief by running cold water over your hands, wrists and inner elbow. A cold cloth on your forehead or the back of your neck can help, too; if you're at home, get into a cold shower and let the water run over you until the heat wave passes.

Hormonal Treatments for Hot Flush Relief

Although medical science continues to study the connection between hormone depletion and hot flushes, hormone replacement therapy – involving oestrogen and/or progesterone – is the most effective medical treatment for vasomotor symptoms known today. Most women find rapid relief from hot flushes once they start taking HRT.

HRT offers a number of other health benefits for women experiencing symptoms of the perimenopause and menopause, including protection against osteoporosis and colorectal cancer. No other treatment for the relief of hot flushes offers the wide-ranging benefits of hormone replacement therapy. Women using oestrogen replacement for the treatment of hot flushes typically experience some relief within a few weeks of beginning treatment, although it may be a month or more before they begin to feel the maximum benefits of the treatment.

Oestrogen is a highly effective tool for combatting symptoms of the perimenopause and menopause, but it's not suitable for all women. See Chapter 11, 'Understanding Hormones and HRT', for more information about the benefits and potential risks of oestrogen.

Oestrogen isn't recommended for women with a personal history of recently diagnosed endometrial cancer. For these women, progestogens have been shown to offer relief from hot flushes. Some recent studies have shown progestogens to decrease hot flushes by as much as 70 to 90 per cent.

Another hormone-based treatment for hot flushes is progesterone cream. This cream, available through prescription, is rubbed on the skin, and the progesterone is slowly absorbed into the woman's system. Although some studies have shown that progesterone cream can offer significant relief from hot flushes, it can be accompanied by some negative side effects, including vaginal bleeding and PMS symptoms such as fatigue.

Only your doctor can help you decide whether or not hormone-based treatments are your best choice for reducing or eliminating hot flushes. If you and your GP decide that hormones aren't right for you, you can choose from other treatment options, including other medications and hormone alternatives, which are discussed in the sections that follow.

Non-hormonal Medications

Though most medical experts prescribe some form of hormone therapy for the relief of vasomotor symptoms accompanying the menopause, these treatments aren't appropriate for all women. Women with active endometrial (uterine) or breast cancers, for example, must usually avoid hormone therapy during cancer treatment. Medical professionals rarely prescribe hormone therapy for women with a personal or family history of blood clotting, liver disease or other conditions that can be triggered or exacerbated by hormone treatments. (See Chapter 11 for more information on hormone replacement therapy.)

To provide relief from hot flushes for women who cannot take oestrogen, medical professionals can prescribe other medications. The following list mentions some of these prescription medications for alleviating hot flushes:

· Clonidine hydrochloride (Dixarit) reduces the responsiveness of the body's vascular system, and has been used for some time in the treatment of high blood pressure. A low dose is used; it may take three to four weeks to begin to see improvement in symptoms; blood pressure must also be monitored. Clonidine has some negative side effects, however: a number of tests have shown that Clonidine can disrupt the sleep of some women. Other side effects reported include dizziness and dry mouth.

· Methyldopa (Aldomet) is another antihypertensive (high blood pressure medication) sometimes used to relieve vasomotor symptoms. Although methyldopa has been shown to reduce the number of hot flushes women experience during the day, it can cause dry mouth, dizziness and headache.

· Selective serotonin reuptake inhibitors (SSRIs), including paroxetine (Seroxat) and venlafaxine (Efexor), are also used to lessen vasomotor symptoms, though doctors don't commonly prescribe them for that purpose. In higher doses, these drugs are used to treat depression. Some tests have shown that relatively low doses of these drugs can reduce the frequency and severity of hot flushes by as much as 50 to 75 per cent, depending upon the specific drug and dosage strategy. Side effects of these drugs include dry mouth, nausea and anxiety.

Many of the non-hormonal treatments for hot flushes and other menopause symptoms are controversial, and their effectiveness, safety and possible side effects and interactions with other medications remain the subject of ongoing studies.

Herbs, Botanicals and Other Alternatives

You need to approach any alternative treatment option with open eyes and healthy scepticism. Botanical extracts, herbal supplements and nutraceutical compounds aren't inspected or approved by the Medicines Control Agency, so they haven't passed the rigorous testing process of approved pharmaceuticals, and they haven't undergone a scientifically controlled process of long-term, in-depth study. Read Chapter 12, 'Alternatives to Hormone Replacement Therapy', for a full discussion of this issue, and be aware that you can't just stroll down the aisle of your local health food shop and choose a safe, effective, natural cure for any of your hormonal symptoms based on the claims of the label (or on other women's experiences you read about in popular consumer magazines or internet chat rooms).

Doctors and scientists around the world, however, continue to evaluate the effectiveness of some of the most popular alternative treatments for the symptoms of the menopause, because many women are choosing to use them. Nevertheless, a great deal remains to be learned about the safety, effectiveness and long-term value of these treatment options.

Some of the alternative treatments most commonly used for the relief of hot flushes include:

- Soya products, including whole soya foods, soya protein capsules and isoflavone extracts, offer some relief from mild hot flushes according to the results of a few studies. Soya proteins are available in soya milk and tofu. Because researchers haven't determined how phytoestrogens in soya interact with cancerous cells, however, these products aren't recommended for women seeking non-hormonal relief from menopause symptoms due to a personal or family history of cancer. Many studies are under way on the use of soya in the treatment of menopause symptoms, so keep watching for new information and ask your doctor about the latest developments.
- Some women have reported that taking vitamin E offered them relief from hot flushes. In studies where participants took a regulated daily dose of 500mg of vitamin E, the women did experience some minor relief (in the order of one less hot flush per day), and the vitamin

caused no negative side effects. At time of writing, no study supports the idea that you can achieve significant relief from hot flushes by taking vitamin E, but (again) studies continue in this area.

Research has not yet determined whether black cohosh is safe for women with breast cancer and other oestrogen-sensitive cancers. If you suspect you may be pregnant, avoid taking black cohosh; it may cause miscarriage or premature birth.

- Black cohosh – derived from the root of a herb – is popular throughout Europe as a treatment for premenstrual syndrome and a number of menopausal symptoms. Although some products containing extracts of black cohosh carry labels that claim they can reduce hot flushes by as much as 25 per cent, many medical experts feel that data to verify the herb's effectiveness is lacking. Black cohosh can have a number of negative side effects, including nausea and dizziness. Avoid black cohosh if you are taking drugs for hypertension: it may intensify the drug's effect of lowering blood pressure. When using black cohosh for the treatment of perimenopause or menopause symptoms, you should limit the total treatment time to no more than six months.

Mind–Body Exercises

Many women have found that they can limit the number and severity of hot flushes using mind–body practices such as yoga, meditation, visualization and deep breathing. Stress, anxiety and fatigue can contribute to the onset and severity of hot flushes; these techniques help calm the mind, relax your muscles and nerves, and keep you feeling rested and at ease. Even when hot flushes do occur, regular practice of these techniques can help you recover more quickly from their effects. And these relaxation techniques and mind–body exercises work to combat a number of other menopausal symptoms, including mood swings, sleeplessness, muscle loss, joint aches and reduced cognitive functions.

tips Use visualization techniques to help cool a hot flush before it builds to a major level. When you feel a hot flush begin to develop, close your eyes and imagine being in a cool, breezy location. Think of the warmth as a liquid, and imagine that you can channel it to flow from your body. Envisage the heat draining out through your hands and feet; as the heat leaves your body, imagine that a cool layer of snow is falling on your head, shoulders and arms.

Use deep breathing to calm a raging hot flush; practise it regularly to help avoid the onset of hot flushes throughout the day and night. Deep, paced breathing is a strong tool for calming the body and the mind – and it's an incredibly easy technique to use. If you feel a hot flush coming on, begin taking deep, slow breaths through your nose. Breathe in to expand your lungs as far as you can, then hold the breath there for a few seconds before you slowly release it. Let your belly swell out and your chest expand as you breathe in, so your body is fully 'inflating' with the breath. When you exhale, empty your lungs completely. Take at least three full, deep breaths and try to remain calm to diminish the hot flush.

A daily programme of meditation and relaxation is a powerful tool for keeping your body calm, focused and strong throughout the day. Its stress-relieving benefits can help ward off hot flushes and other stress-related symptoms of the menopause. A ten-minute relaxation session is easy to fit into your morning and evening schedule, and it's easy to do.

Sit or lie down in a quiet place with your eyes closed. Consciously relax every muscle in your body, beginning with your feet and continuing the relaxation up toward your head. Concentrate on a single word or object that has personal meaning for you; if other ideas, worries or mental chatter enter your mind, dismiss them and return to the thought of your focus word. After ten minutes open your eyes, remain seated and take three deep breaths before continuing with your day.

Yoga is an excellent practice for increasing flexibility, building muscle strength and endurance, and eliminating the negative effects of stress on your body. Practising yoga stretches for 20 to 30 minutes three times a week can help reduce the negative effects of stress on your body, as it stretches your muscles, improves your balance and encourages deep, full breathing. Regular yoga practice can also help reduce insomnia, so you fall asleep faster and stay asleep longer. All these benefits can help eliminate the anxiety triggers that can contribute to hot flushes.

CHAPTER 17

Finding Your New Sexuality

Among the many changes you may experience in the perimenopause and menopause are a changing sexual attitude and appetite. Your age and hormone levels don't determine your sexuality; you are who you have always been, and your fundamental feelings and attitudes about sex don't change when you stop ovulating. But the physical and emotional evolution of a maturing mind and body can colour your sexual response.

Checking Your Sexual Attitude

Your attitudes about sex and your own sexuality today are greatly influenced by the attitudes you had about these issues when you were younger. If you enjoyed sex and expected to be sexually satisfied when you were 30, you're more likely to continue to enjoy sex as you move through your 50s and beyond. Nevertheless, some women report a declining interest in sex after the menopause, and most experts agree that changes in attitude accompanied by changes in physical health can play a strong role in that shift.

Here are some common reasons women may experience a decline in sexual interest:

- Painful intercourse, resulting from vaginal dryness
- Lack of a partner or a partner's declining ability to satisfy
- Feelings of low self-esteem or physical undesirability
- Feeling too tired, too busy or otherwise preoccupied to enjoy sexual activity

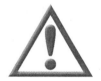

Don't let illness, side effects of medication or a reluctance to discuss sexual issues with your doctor stand in the way of your ability to enjoy an active sex life. Talk to your doctor about changes in your sexual ability or desire. Maintaining your sexual health is important to your overall physical and emotional well-being.

Every woman has unique sexual needs and interests, and many women (and men) have a limited sexual desire at some point in their lives. But if you find your interest in sex waning – at any age – it's important for you to understand why. Maintaining and nurturing your sexuality is important for your physical and emotional health. You shouldn't expect to stop enjoying sex as you age. It's well worth your time to take steps to keep your sex drive alive and thriving through the menopause and beyond it.

Overcoming Physical Barriers

If you don't feel physically fit and healthy, you're less likely to enjoy an active, healthy sex life. Although you can't postpone the menopause or the effects of ageing indefinitely, you don't have to let some of the physical symptoms of the menopause prevent you from remaining sexually active. If physical problems are interfering with your sexual desire or ability – from vaginal dryness or stress incontinence to fatigue resulting from sleep disturbances, illness or medication – the first step toward resolving those problems is to talk to your GP, who may refer you to a gynaecologist. Your doctor can recommend treatment options, exercise, dietary or medication changes or other therapeutic solutions that can lessen or even resolve your physical barriers to an enjoyable sex life. And, as with all aspects of your health care, you may be able to improve your sexual health through some changes in your lifestyle choices.

The Basics

Your daily practices play a big role in your overall fitness – you know that. The same stresses, habits and substances that damage other aspects of your health can limit your desire and ability to enjoy sex as well. Here are some basics for maintaining your sexual fitness:

- **Eat properly and exercise regularly:** Nutrition and exercise are critical to your overall health as you age, and they play an important role in preserving your sexual health. Regular aerobic, weight-bearing and stretching exercises keep your body feeling active and alive. Middle age weight gain and ebbing muscle strength and endurance can erode your sexual desire. When your body is strong and fit, you're more energetic and you take a greater interest in all aspects of your life – including sex. If your body is strong and healthy, you're less likely to think of it as an ageing relic, and you're more likely to enjoy sharing it with a partner. Also exercise releases endorphins, the 'feel happy' neurotransmitters in your brain. If you feel better about your body, you're more likely to feel good about sharing it with someone physically. Read Chapters 13, 'Eating for a Healthy Menopause', and

14, 'Building Exercise into Your Menopause Plan', for diet and exercise ideas.

- **Rest and manage stress:** If your daily routine is too overwhelming to allow you to enjoy an active sex life, it's probably damaging your health in other ways. Stress can lead to headaches, indigestion, muscle pain, depression and – not surprisingly – a diminished desire for and response to sexual activity. Try to learn what's causing your stress, then do what you can to avoid the stressors. Talk to family and friends, remember to exercise regularly, and learn and practise regular relaxation techniques.

- **Cut down on alcohol and stop smoking:** Most medical experts agree that one or two alcoholic drinks a day aren't bad for your health (unless you have conditions or are taking medication that precludes the use of any alcohol). But drinking too much alcohol can lead to depression, weight gain and – in some cases – an increased stress response. Smoking fuels stress as well, and it saps your body of strength and energy. All of these effects can erode your interest in sexual activity and dampen your response to sexual stimulation.

Exercise offers a number of benefits for women at any age, but did you know that it could give you a real sexual boost? Some studies have shown that people who practise some form of regular exercise achieve orgasm more easily than do people who don't exercise at all.

- **Treat vaginal dryness:** If you suffer from vaginal dryness, intercourse can be painful. Oestrogen replacement can help relieve vaginal dryness and keep vaginal tissues moist, elastic and healthy (see Chapter 11 for more information on the benefits and risks of HRT). Women who cannot use hormone replacement therapy (such as a woman with a history of breast cancer) now have newer options available, such as oestrogen suppositories: Vagifem vaginal tablets contain the active ingredient estradiol (previously spelt oestradiol), a naturally occurring form of the main female sex hormone, oestrogen. The tablets release small amounts of estradiol into the vagina. They are used on a short-term basis to help return the vaginal tissues to normal and relieve the soreness and irritation of the vagina.

Improve Sexual Response with Pelvic Floor Exercises

You've probably heard of the pelvic floor (or Kegel) exercises; many women use them to return the strength and condition of their vaginal muscles after childbirth. Other women use the exercises to improve their ability to control stress incontinence, a problem that many women develop as they approach the menopause. The technique has also been shown to offer women another important benefit: strengthening vaginal muscles can increase sexual health and pleasure.

The exercises strengthen the pelvic floor muscles that extend from the pubic bone to the coccyx and surround your vaginal opening and the opening to your urinary tract. Strengthening these muscles enables you to contract your vaginal opening, increasing the amount and intensity of the contact between your vagina and your partner's penis. The exercises also increase the blood flow to (and the sensitivity of) your genital area. Practising them regularly can increase the physical sensations of intercourse, making sex more pleasurable for you and your partner.

Los Angeles obstetrician/gynaecologist Arnold Kegel developed the exercises named for him in the mid-1940s as a non-surgical solution for his patients who were battling incontinence. He later realized that the exercises helped new mothers recover from the physical effects of labour and vaginal childbirth. Today, many women do pelvic floor exercises to make their vaginal muscles stronger and more resilient in preparation for childbirth.

You can identify the relevant muscles the next time you urinate. When you begin urinating, squeeze your muscles to stop the flow. Try to start and stop the flow several times in the same sitting. The muscles you're contracting are those of your pelvic floor musculature – the same set of muscles that you exercise with the exercises. Once you learn to identify and contract that muscle, you can do your exercises anywhere – but don't do them while urinating, as this is bad for your bladder. Just contract the pelvic floor muscle and hold it for a count of five. Breathe normally and repeat the contraction, hold, and release ten times. Do this exercise every day – do a dozen repetitions when you're sitting and waiting for a red light to change, or when you're on hold during a phone call. After a month or two of practice, you should notice that you have more control over your bladder and some improved sensation during sexual activity (including masturbation).

Enjoying Your Body

If you lead a hectic life, filled with the responsibilities of work, home and family, you may have little time to think about yourself – your body, your mind, your pleasure. As your body begins to change with age, it's easy to begin to think of it as your enemy. Something you've always depended on (although you may not have lavished much attention on it) is letting you down just when you need it most. Many women simply lose touch with their physicality, choosing to ignore their physical condition and respond in the out-of-sight-out-of-mind approach we all know so well.

A multivitamin-mineral supplement may be an easy and inexpensive way to promote your sexuality – and your general health. Vitamin E has been shown in some studies to increase sexual desire, and zinc may help foster sexual arousal (oysters are high in zinc). Selenium is another mineral that is the subject of ongoing studies of sexuality.

The truth is that your body matters; your physical needs matter, too. If you find yourself looking at your body with disappointment or wanting to ignore your body and its physical condition and needs, take conscious action to overcome those feelings. Your body is yours for life, and keeping it healthy, vital and fit as you approach the menopause has never been more important.

All this book's recommendations for exercise, health care, regular check-ups, relaxation techniques, hair and skin treatments and good diet have been aimed at the important goal of taking care of your body so you can enjoy it. Spending time caring for your body will encourage you to take pleasure in its strength and capabilities. By feeling confident and at ease about your body, you're more likely to enjoy the pleasures of its sexual responses. Humans are sexual beings, and sexual enjoyment is good for both the body and the mind.

Explore your sexual interests and fantasies. Don't feel ashamed of your sexual orientation, desires or needs. Many doctors and sex therapists encourage their patients to masturbate to increase their ability to respond to sexual stimulation and to combat stress and anxiety. If you'd like more information on how to become aroused and stay stimulated (by yourself or with a partner), visit your local bookshop, which is full of self-help books on improving your sexual response – or visit an online bookshop such as *Amazon.co.uk* if you feel embarrassed at buying such books over the counter. Even reading a steamy novel can help you to become aroused, or hire a video with some love scenes featuring a favourite film star. You don't have to turn to pornography – just allow yourself to explore and enjoy the sexual arousal you might normally hold back.

Take Your Partner Along for the Ride

If you are in a committed relationship as you near midlife, the chances are strong that your partner in that relationship is ageing, too. His or her sexual performance and desire may be suffering as much – or even more – than your own. If you and your partner experience a decline in sexual intimacy, you should talk about it.

Many couples ignore sexual problems because they're too embarrassed to discuss them together – let alone with a doctor. But most sexual issues don't resolve themselves. Even if you take action to improve your own sexual response and desire, your partner may not benefit from it. Some men and women can feel a bit overwhelmed by their partner's increased sexual desire, so talking with your partner is your first step to getting your sex life back on track.

If your partner is suffering from physical problems that are affecting his or her sexual performance, talking with a doctor is the next step. A GP or gynaecologist may decide to refer you to a sex therapist if your condition warrants it. Keep an open mind and follow your doctor's recommendations. Maintaining the health of your sexual relationship is an important part of remaining healthy and happy together.

As he ages, your male partner may need more stimulation in order to achieve an erection. As you're learning to enjoy your sexuality more, don't forget to pay attention to your partner's needs. Many couples find that as their sexual relationship matures they draw increasing pleasure from the non-intercourse parts of their lovemaking, and use their hands and mouths more frequently during sex.

Enhancing Your Sexual Experience

You may find that your lovemaking simply needs some new life. Take this opportunity to enjoy a second 'first romance' with your partner. Learn to touch each other again and take pleasure in your physical contact; take baths and showers together and spend more time in touching and foreplay during lovemaking. Let your partner know what feels good to you and find out what he or she enjoys most, and explore your fantasies. Don't forget to use vaginal creams and lubricants to make the sexual experience more enjoyable. (If you're using condoms, remember to use water-based lubricants; petroleum can weaken the condom wall and cause breaks and tears.) At this stage in your life, you can move beyond the shyness and embarrassment of adolescence. Your bodies are yours to enjoy, so don't hold back.

Be Creative

Don't become complacent about your sex life. Many women expect spontaneous bursts of admiration from their partners, even if they haven't been demonstrating much interest in their body or their sexuality lately. If you've stopped paying attention to your physical appearance, take some time to do the things that will make you look and feel more beautiful. Get a new haircut or have a facial. Stop at the cosmetics counter at your local department store, and ask for some ideas for revitalizing your appearance. When you look better, you feel more sexually appealing.

If you're having sex with more than one partner, don't forget to be scrupulously clean and use condoms for protection from sexually transmitted diseases. And if you haven't gone at least 12 months without a period (or were diagnosed as menopausal through a blood test), you can still be fertile, so use appropriate birth-control measures.

Would a new nightgown or dressing gown make you feel sexier? Silky, flattering lingerie comes in a variety of styles and sizes, so visit a lingerie store to check out your options. If you've grown self-conscious about your midlife physique, wearing a flattering negligee during lovemaking can help you feel more confident and relaxed. And while you're there, try some of the new bust-shaping bras. Many women in midlife have a cleavage for the first time, so why not take advantage of it?

Setting the mood is all-important for revitalizing your lovemaking. Lower the lights, burn some aromatic candles and play some soft, sensual music. Now is the time to relax and explore sensual pleasures. Put away the tracksuit, and dress for dinner. Use your imagination and have fun with sex. Be creative, experiment and try to be open with your partner about your feelings and responses to whatever you experience together.

CHAPTER 18

Overcoming Mood Swings, Anxiety and Depression

Many women do experience depression, anxiety and/or mood swings during the perimenopause. Mood disorders can be triggered by a number of causes, and if you suffer from them – at any time in your life – it's important that you understand the source of your problems as well as how to treat them. Through medical treatment, stress management and wise lifestyle choices, you can learn to regain control of your emotional stability.

Looking Stress in the Eye

Stress is a fact of life for everyone, and women approaching the age of the menopause certainly aren't immune from its effects. In fact, women in the perimenopause may be more susceptible to the health-damaging side effects of stress than they have been at previous times in their lives. Stress exacerbates a wide range of medical problems, from stomach disorders and headaches to insomnia and even depression. Stress can be a major contributor to mood swings, anxiety and mild depression, so if you suffer from these emotional disorders, one of your first steps towards recovery may be to identify the sources of stress in your life.

Women in midlife can be faced with any number of stressors, including career and financial issues, body image changes, emerging health problems, divorce, widowhood, struggles with teenage children and increasing responsibilities for ageing parents. Although many women will have dealt with some or all of these issues at previous times in life, the added stress of adjusting to hormonal fluctuations, hot flushes, weight gain or other potential side effects of the perimenopause can make stress even harder to bear during midlife.

Learn to delegate responsibilities; if you do this early, before the pressure really builds up, you're less likely to crack.

Some of the most common symptoms of stress include headaches, sleeplessness, indigestion, forgetfulness, an inability to concentrate and ongoing feelings of anger and unhappiness. Stress can leave you feeling drained of all good feeling, and it can lead to overeating, drinking too much alcohol or stepping up the pace of other unhealthy stress habits such as cigarette smoking. If you experience any of these symptoms of stress, you need to realize that you have a real, health-threatening problem and take action to determine its sources and potential solutions. Unless you find ways to eliminate or manage stress, you won't be successful in combatting the mood-related problems you may experience during the perimenopause.

Managing Stress

You can't avoid all sources of stress, but you may be able to find ways to work around many of them. For example, if a hectic work and family schedule is depleting your energy and contributing to stress, try to see what activities you can trim from your list of daily activities. Can you ask a partner for help in managing household tasks or running errands? Can you afford to hire a service to do the laundry, pick up and deliver dry cleaning or take over major cleaning jobs around the house? If you have children, can you ask them to step up their helping and take more responsibility for their own needs, or to help more around the house? If ageing parents are presenting increasing demands on your time, can you get any type of community support assistance, such as meal deliveries or the services of a visiting nurse?

And don't stop at examining your home and family responsibilities, either. Evaluate your job and work habits to try to spot stress fixes there, as well. Can you ask your boss for flexible work times, so you can schedule your commute when traffic is less hectic, or even arrange to work at home one day a week? Can you find someone to share a car with? If you commute by train, can you do some of your work on a laptop computer and save time at the office? If you have problems with a colleague, can you schedule a meeting to try to resolve the issues, or at least to lessen the tension? Can a personal organizer, meeting scheduler programme or other software help you save time and cut down on unnecessary panic and last-minute emergencies? Can you ask a well-organized colleague for help in finding ways to trim the fat from your work habits?

fact Don't assume that you absolutely *must* or *can't* do anything. This isn't a time to mindlessly adhere to old routines or to be driven by false necessity; rethink your priorities and learn to devote your time and attention to the things that serve you best.

When you've pinpointed and reduced the stressors that you can, find ways to cope with the stress you can't get rid of. Exercise regularly, spend time engaged in leisure activities you enjoy, eat a healthy diet and go easy on your mind and body – don't expect to perform every task flawlessly and on time.

Whatever the possible solutions, the first key to relieving stress is to come to grips with the fact that stress presents a real health risk – one you simply cannot overlook. Stress will wear you out, age your body and mind, drain your spirit and cause serious and lasting health problems. Although you may feel that you have no options – that you're stuck with the stressful situations you currently endure – you do have options available to you. Talk to your doctor, a therapist, a counsellor, a friend, a minister or a trusted family member, and ask for help in finding ways to manage stress.

Your stress may be connected to a medical condition or the medication or treatment you're using to combat one. Your doctor may be able to adjust your medication or offer additional treatment options that can help you reduce and manage any health-related stressors you're encountering.

Recognize the Symptoms

Nearly 25 per cent of all women suffer from some form of depression at some time during their lives. Many studies have shown that women first experience depression when they're in their 20s, or even younger. And although the menopause doesn't automatically signal the onset of depression, women who have suffered from depression earlier in life, or women who have had postpartum depression or even severe premenstrual syndrome (PMS), are more likely to have recurring depression during perimenopause. Women who have a family history of depression also run more risk of suffering from depression during the perimenopause.

Many researchers believe that the physical changes of the perimenopause – the fluctuating levels of oestrogen and progesterone many women experience during this time – can contribute to mood swings and other emotional symptoms of the perimenopause, although the mechanisms of their impact are under continual study. Doctors know, however, that oestrogen is directly related to our body's production of serotonin – an important chemical that works in the brain to regulate moods. As oestrogen levels shift, so does the brain's supply of serotonin – and therefore moods can shift as well.

Body chemistry isn't the only thing that can trigger midlife mood decay. Women who are dealing with changing roles at home or at work, changing levels of energy, or diminishing feelings of general fitness and well-being are at risk of suffering from emotional upheavals and imbalances.

> **tips**
>
> As you move into the perimenopause, it's important that you remain aware of your feelings and alert for signs of emotional problems. Just as you have to check up on and monitor your physical health regularly, you need to watch for and deal with symptoms of emotional disorder to maintain your overall fitness and well-being.

Coming to grips with your emotional upsets by recognizing symptoms and tracking them to their source can be a first step towards resolving the problem. When you have some understanding of the types and severity of the symptoms you're experiencing, you're able to determine your next course of action better. You may be able to control mild mood disturbances simply by changing your diet, exercise programme or reactions to certain stress-inducing stimuli. Such techniques are covered later in this chapter, along with information about medication, counselling and other treatment options that can help restore emotional order and balance when lifestyle and behavioural changes aren't enough.

Tracking Your Mood Swings

Mood shifts are relatively mild changes in mood that can quickly take a woman from feelings of joy to anger, fatigue or despair. The triggers for these responses can be unpredictable – and sometimes seemingly inconsequential. Perimenopausal women who report mood swings cite a wide range of stimuli for these events. If you're swinging, you can be moved to tears by a song on the radio or the colour of the light as evening falls over your back garden. You can become incredibly angry when a colleague asks for clarification of a point you made in a memo, when children or a partner fail to take care of their household responsibilities, or when you forget to stop and pick up the dry cleaning on your way home. Mood swings can sometimes be no more than a normal response magnified to a level much higher than normal.

During the perimenopause, mood swings simply indicate that your body and mind are adjusting to a variety of physical, emotional and social changes that accompany this phase of your life. Although it's easy to dismiss these emotions as being 'just the change', don't fail to recognize them as your response to some real experience or stimulus.

You may be reacting to some source of irritation, unhappiness, discomfort, fear, love, joy or longing. As oestrogen levels rise and fall due to your body's release of the hormone, serotonin levels can rise and fall, too, taking your mood right along with them. Alternatively, mood swings can be a response to a medical condition or chemical imbalance in your body – one, perhaps, that can be treated through counselling, medication or other therapy. Your mood swings can teach you a lot about who you are, what issues and changes you're dealing with, and where you want to go during this transition in your life.

You can expect some mood swings in your life, especially as you reach midlife. But many women in the perimenopause develop mood swings that interfere with their lives. Frequent or severe mood swings can create problems with family, colleagues and friends; cause days off work; discourage participation in social functions or enjoyable activities; or create feelings of alienation, exhaustion, fear and a lack of control. If mood swings are severe or frequent enough to get in the way of your full – and fulfilling – life, take action to bring them under control.

The Symptoms of Anxiety

Anxiety is a natural, healthy response to certain realities of life – beginning a new job, meeting upcoming deadlines, passing examinations and so on. But anxiety that interferes with your ability to function at full capacity throughout your day and then sleep soundly throughout the night is definitely unhealthy. Anxiety can be a side effect of a more serious mood-destabilizing condition – depression.

Anxiety can be associated with depression, or it can be a side effect of sleeplessness, excess fatigue or unmanageable levels of stress. Many people suffering from anxiety describe it as overwhelming feelings of fear, nervousness or the conviction that something dreadful is about to happen – although they often can't pinpoint what that something may be. When these feelings begin to interfere with normal, everyday functioning, they may represent an anxiety disorder. Some other symptoms of anxiety include:

· An unshakeable feeling of fear, dread or worry that lasts for more than three days
· Chest pain, racing heart or fast breathing
· Stomach pain, cramp or diarrhoea
· Hand-wringing, pacing or other repetitive nervous movements

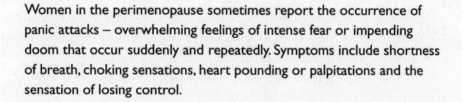

Women in the perimenopause sometimes report the occurrence of panic attacks – overwhelming feelings of intense fear or impending doom that occur suddenly and repeatedly. Symptoms include shortness of breath, choking sensations, heart pounding or palpitations and the sensation of losing control.

Anxiety that goes unchecked can develop into anxiety disorders. These disorders include social phobias, such as agoraphobia (fear of going out in public), specific phobias (such as fear of dogs or spiders) or obsessive behaviour (such as obsessive hand washing or repeatedly checking door locks or appliance switches).

Know the Symptoms of Depression

Although transient feelings of sadness, despair or general dissatisfaction with life are common during the perimenopause, if these feelings are long-lasting or severe they could be signalling the onset of depression. Insomnia, fatigue, hot flushes and other perimenopausal symptoms can trigger minor mood disorders during the perimenopause. But major depression goes well beyond the typical reaction to these perimenopausal symptoms. Although sometimes doctors can't identify the cause, major depression is often the result of a biological or chemical imbalance that requires careful diagnosis and treatment.

Researchers in the USA have found that women are more likely than men to increase their consumption of alcohol when depressed. Abusing alcohol or drugs compounds the problems of midlife, and women in the perimenopause should be wary of self-medicating with these substances.

Sometimes depression itself can be a symptom or side effect of some major life event, such as a divorce, the death of a loved one, losing a job or dealing with a severe or ongoing medical problem – all problems that can occur to women at midlife. But these sorts of event-triggered depressions may pass with time or resolve themselves quickly, without the need for special treatment or therapy. Sometimes, however, these events can lead to depression that deepens into a deeper depression that women are unlikely to overcome without some form of treatment.

The characteristic symptoms of clinical depression follow:

· Feelings of hopelessness, worthlessness or guilt, or a general depressed mood that lasts most of the day, nearly every day for two weeks or longer
· Fatigue and loss of energy
· Difficulty concentrating
· Loss of interest in activities you previously found to be pleasurable
· Sleep disorder, whether sleeping too much or suffering from insomnia
· Recurrent thoughts of suicide or death

Major depression is an illness, with many options for treatment. If you suffer from depression, the sooner you get help, the more quickly and effectively you can overcome the physical and emotional side effects of this devastating condition.

> Depression can harm you, your family, your job and your friends and colleagues. Those around you are likely to be confused, saddened, worried or even irritated by your depressed behaviour. Don't let your depression become 'contagious'; talk to a health professional to get the help you need.

Take Action

You may have difficulty recognizing that you are suffering from an emotional imbalance or mood disorder. Many women can go through months of emotional turmoil thinking, 'It's just a bad day', then 'What a bad week', then 'This month has been awful', and still believe that they're just feeling temporarily down, moody or out of sorts. Often these women are taken aback when a friend, partner or relative expresses concerns over their moodiness, irritability or remoteness.

If you or those around you suspect that your emotional behaviour may signal a mood disorder, you need to take action to seek a diagnosis and, if necessary, make behavioural changes or begin treatment. Your goal is to get your life back in balance, so you can regain your sense of confidence and purpose.

Rule Out Medical Causes

Mood swings, depression and anxiety can be triggered or made worse by medical problems. Thyroid disorders can sometimes result in depression, as can the use of some medications used to treat hypertension. Some weight-loss drugs can trigger a rise in anxiety levels or even panic attacks. As you seek to find the causes and solutions for your emotional imbalances, begin by talking with your gynaecologist or GP. That individual can review your medications and health history to uncover any potential medical causes for your mood disorders.

Your doctor can also uncover contributing medical conditions, such as insomnia, sleep apnoea or extreme hormonal imbalances, that may contribute to your mood swings. If your doctor uncovers specific medical causes for your condition, he or she can adjust your medication, treat the contributing medical condition or suggest other specific treatment options best suited to resolving those issues.

Explore Your Treatment Options

When medical complications have been ruled out, you have several treatment options available to you for diminishing – or even eliminating – your mood disorder symptoms. The option that's best for you is determined, in part, by the severity of your problem and your personal and family medical history.

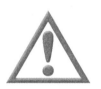

Stress can trigger the biological changes that accompany depression, and it appears that hormonal shifts can trigger those changes, too. That's why women with a family or personal history of depression must be particularly careful to monitor and manage stress as they approach the age of the menopause.

If you suffer from clinical depression, your doctor is likely to prescribe some sort of antidepressant medication. (See the section 'For Combatting Insomnia, Depression and Anxiety' in Chapter 12.) Following is a quick list of some of the most commonly prescribed antidepressant and antianxiety medications:

- Selective serotonin reuptake inhibitors (SSRIs), including fluoxetine, sertraline and paroxetine (marketed as Prozac, Lustral and Seroxat). Although SSRIs can cause depressed sexual response and other side effects in certain individuals, they are non-addictive and work by helping your body make better use of the serotonin it naturally produces. Fluoxetine is also approved for premenstrual dysphoric disorder (PMDD) and is available as a once-a-week timed-release dosage.

· Antianxiety drugs, or anxiolytics such as buspirone, can lessen the effects of depression, anxiety and sleeplessness, and they also can treat the symptoms of PMDD that many perimenopausal women experience as they move closer to the menopause. Anxiolytics can have a slightly sedative effect, so many doctors prescribe them for short periods of time only.

> **tips**
>
> Many doctors prescribe antidepressants in combination with hormone replacement therapy for perimenopausal or menopausal women with severe depression. Although HRT is rarely the first-course treatment for depression, it can alleviate symptoms such as hot flushes and insomnia that contribute to depression, and it offers other benefits for menopausal women. (See Chapter 11 for more information.)

Psychological counselling – psychotherapy – is a powerful treatment option for women experiencing excess anxiety, stress or mood disturbance during the perimenopause and menopause. Most studies have shown that counselling in conjunction with antidepressant medication offers more long-term and effective results than does a treatment using medication alone. Though you may not experience the benefits of psychotherapy immediately after you begin treatment, its effects can be long-lasting and wide-reaching.

The two types of psychotherapy you are most likely to receive for emotional problems associated with the perimenopause are interpersonal therapy or cognitive-behavioural therapy. Interpersonal therapy explores the relationships in your life and how they may be contributing to your emotional problems. This type of therapy also teaches you how you may use the strength and support you gain from your relationships to help deal with emotional issues.

Cognitive-behavioural therapy examines your core thoughts and beliefs and how they determine your actions in response to life. If you have developed a pessimistic or negative attitude towards life in general, this type of therapy can help you see the world in a more balanced perspective and learn more effective ways of viewing and coping with life.

Learning to be optimistic can have real physical and emotional health benefits. Although no conclusive studies have proven the benefits of optimism, many medical professionals have observed that their pessimistic patients are prone to have elevated blood pressure, less resistance to disease and a slower recovery time following illnesses or injury.

Staying 'On the Level'

If you are experiencing mild mood disturbances, anxiety or general but recurring feelings of the blues, you have a number of simple self-treatment options for levelling out the emotional roller-coaster ride.

First, give your body and mind healthy amounts of good fuel, activity and rest. Eat a healthy diet that emphasizes fruit, vegetables and whole grains and skips high-fat, low-nutrient foods loaded with sugar, salt and simple carbohydrates. Limiting the amount of caffeine, salt, MSG and sugar you consume can help your body remain active and alert, rather than jumpy and fatigued. Your physical and emotional health are inextricably linked, and you can't maintain either with an unhealthy diet.

Here are some other good guidelines to follow:

- **Eat sensible amounts of food throughout the day.** If you stuff yourself or try to eat your way out of a low mood, you just add to the problem by contributing to weight gain, low self-esteem and poor body image. But if you skip meals or rely on junk food or fast-food fixes because you're just too busy to worry about when and what you're eating, you can stress both your body and mind – and rob them of the nutrients they need. If a lack of time is a problem, check out the frozen foods section of your local supermarket. Lots of frozen meals are tasty, nutritious and low in fat and calories. Bad nutrition can lead to illness, fatigue and a host of other problems that can leave you feeling hopeless and depressed. Caring about your body is essential to caring for your mind.

· **Be active.** Although mood swings, anxiety and depression can leave you feeling frozen – uninterested in life and incapable of doing anything to participate in it – activity is one of the best ways to lift and stabilize your mood. Physical activity triggers your body to releases mood-lifting endorphins, and it gets your heart pumping to circulate healthy, oxygenated blood throughout your body. Participating in activities with family and friends can help lighten your mood, broaden your perspective on the issues that are troubling you and renew your hopes and interests so you can deal more effectively with issues that threaten your emotional health. Get involved in activities that challenge both mind and body; pick up a hobby or revisit old interests that engage your creativity and motivate you to exercise your talents. Physical activity and regular exercise actually leave you feeling more energetic.

· **Practice meditation or relaxation techniques.** Meditation, relaxation techniques and mind–body exercises such as yoga and t'ai chi are powerful tools for relieving hot flushes and other symptoms of stress, anxiety and mild depression. (See the section on 'Mind–Body Exercises' in Chapter 16 for more information on these techniques.) Fifteen-minute sessions of meditation, deep breathing or relaxation every morning and evening can help reduce or even eliminate much of the stress and mood-altering emotional upheavals of the perimenopause.

· **Get plenty of rest.** Try to establish and maintain a regular sleep schedule in which you go to sleep and rise at the same times every day – including at weekends. Take time to read, listen to music or soak in a hot bath to relax and prepare yourself for sleep. Don't exercise or eat large amounts of food late in the evening.

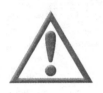

If you find yourself waking and unable to return to sleep early in the morning for more than three or four days in a row, you should contact your doctor. Re-establishing a healthy sleep pattern is essential to maintaining good health; the longer your sleep is disturbed, the more difficulty you'll have returning to a normal cycle.

You Don't Have to Do It Alone

No one treatment option is right – or even effective – for every woman. But any woman suffering from mood disorders should talk with a doctor, counsellor, mentor or other trusted adviser to discuss all appropriate treatments. Depression and other mood disturbances are not a typical by-product of the ageing process. A willingness to admit and discuss mood disorders is your best weapon for overcoming them.

Though women are statistically more likely than men to suffer from depression, they are also more likely to look for help in overcoming issues that affect their emotional health. Your friends, family, colleagues, doctor, minister or other counsellors can help you find ways to put emotional issues to rest, so you can concentrate on becoming healthier, stronger and more engaged in life as each year passes.

CHAPTER 19

Keeping
Your Mind Sharp

With our bodies living longer than at any time in history, our surest chance for a happy and independent old age lies in keeping our minds as finely tuned and functional as possible – for as long as we possibly can.

How Your Brain Changes as You Age

Most medical and scientific authorities agree that the mind's ability to think clearly and quickly changes with age, but those changes aren't linked to the menopause. The brain doesn't have a 'use by' shelf life exactly; most nerves are capable of lasting for a hundred years or more. But changes in the brain's physical size and functions do occur with age, and those changes can have an impact on how well you can recall information stored in your brain.

The human brain shrinks slightly after the age of 50 as a result of a loss of water content. The shrinkage itself doesn't impair your memory, but the loss of frontal-lobe volume that accompanies that loss can. Some neuroscientists believe frontal lobes can shrink up to 30 per cent between the ages of 50 and 90. Frontal lobes are critical to complex thinking – your ability to reason, pay attention and perform multiple tasks at the same time. A diminished capacity in your frontal lobes can diminish your abilities in all of these cognitive functions.

Perhaps most important to preserving memory and recall is the brain's hippocampus – the part of the brain where memory is stored, created and retrieved. Some researchers believe the hippocampus can lose ability with age – resulting in a slowing down of the brain's ability to store and retrieve memory. Exacerbating this slowdown are metabolic changes and a dwindling number of dendrites – the neurons that transmit the brain's signals. All of these changes can combine to make your brain feel duller and slower.

You don't need to panic that you're suffering an onset of early Alzheimer's disease every time you misplace your car keys – especially not as you approach the age of the menopause. Many of the symptoms of the menopause, including mood swings, sleeplessness, increased susceptibility to stress and fluctuating levels of hormones, can contribute to less efficient cognitive functions – but most of these symptoms are relatively mild and transient.

Take Steps to Keep Your Mind Sharp

You have a number of options available to you for keeping your brain functioning as strongly as possible into and through the menopause. However, maintaining good cognitive functions takes effort. You can't just take a pill or wear a special bracelet to protect your brain's functions. The first step toward maintaining a healthy, active brain is to maintain a healthy, active body. That requires good nutrition (including proper nutritional supplements) and regular exercise.

Experts agree that all individuals aged 50 and over are wise to take steps to preserve their cognitive strength. Even at advanced ages the mind continues to be capable of learning and recalling new information – but this type of mental fitness requires effort.

Give Your Brain the Nutrition It Needs

Your brain needs fuel in order to function. Experts estimate that the brain uses 20 per cent or more of the body's energy. Glucose and antioxidants are important components of your brain's nutrition, so make sure your diet includes plenty of whole grains, fruit and vegetables. The brain also may benefit from folates – found in leafy green vegetables, lentils and other legumes. Folic acid, a laboratory-produced version of folate, is included in many multivitamins and some fortified foods. Studies also show that daily recommended doses of vitamin E and selenium may help slow the diminishment of cognitive functions. Recently, Alpha-Lipoic acid and Coenzyme Q_{10} have been recognized to improve brain health, cognitive function and memory.

Doctors have found that oestrogen helps aid the brain's functions of remembering and storing new information, so oestrogen therapy can help to postpone a decline in cognitive functions and protect short-term and long-term memory. Oestrogen also helps to improve the circulation to the brain by directly dilating the critical blood vessels involved. If you are receiving HRT as part of your general menopausal health maintenance plan, you can add this benefit to the many others you'll receive from that therapy.

Exercise Your Body to Keep Your Brain Healthy

Regular exercise – at least 20 minutes a day, but 30 minutes to an hour daily is best – is one great way to preserve your mental acuity. Aerobic exercise helps get the blood coursing through your system, carrying oxygen and glucose to your brain – two substances the brain needs in order to function.

Regular exercise also can prod the brain into producing more molecules that help protect and produce the brain's neurons. Although studies are still underway to establish the link between exercise and increased brain neurons, many researchers – including those involved with Alzheimer's disease research – are studying the protective effects of regular physical exercise on the brain's neural paths for transmitting signals.

Physical exercise is a great way to reduce stress, and stress can take a serious toll on cognitive functions. Stress inhibits your ability to concentrate, and it can shorten your lifespan. In the USA, the New England Centenarian Study found that one trait common among those who live beyond the age of 100 is an ability to handle stress. (See Chapter 18 for other recommended stress-busters.)

Exercise Your Brain to Keep It Lively

Some simple, but effective, techniques for putting your mind through some hoops to keep it active and highly functional are presented later in this chapter. But many of the most important things you can do to hone your memory are really just good habits – things you do every day as a matter of course that keep your brain's neurons charged and firing, and your hippocampus fully loaded and ready to dispense information.

Mental exercise can increase the size of different areas of the brain, just as physical exercise increases muscle size. Researchers have long known that musicians' brains are different in proportion than those of non-musicians, but a study of the brains of London taxi drivers, reported in March 2000, indicated that this effect can continue into late adulthood. London cabbies are required to spend two years memorizing all the main streets, back alleys, shops and businesses in London – information known as 'the Knowledge' – and then pass a memory test to get their licences. Researchers found that the brain of a trained and licensed cabbie had a hippocampus larger than that area in the brains of a control group. And the hippocampus continued to enlarge as the cabbie used the Knowledge. Cabbies who had been driving for some time – some for over 40 years – had a larger hippocampus than their less-experienced colleagues.

When you're trying to memorize or recall something important, eliminate all other distractions. Turn off the television, lower the volume on the stereo and go to a quiet place where people aren't chattering around you. You'll find you have to put in less time and effort if you are able to concentrate better, and you'll retain the information longer.

You don't have to build a street map of London in your brain to improve your memory. But you do have to make some effort to boost your memory. Here are some basic brain-building practices:

Pay attention: The first clue to preserving – or even improving – your memory is to learn to pay attention to what is being said and what is happening around you. Many researchers believe that inattentiveness is a major cause of forgetfulness in people of any age. If you don't learn how to really listen and observe, your brain has no opportunity to absorb and store information. And pay attention to your actions as well; the classic lost-keys problem is easily resolved by creating a place in the home where you always put your keys, for example. Write out lists of important things you must do, and read the list out loud as you think about each item and visualize some image or action that each represents to you.

Slow down and repeat information: When you hear a new name or have to commit a list of things to memory, stop, slow down and repeat the information you have to remember several times. Repeat the name to yourself (other word-association ideas for remembering names appear in the following text), and – if you've just met someone – repeat that person's name during the conversation, as in, 'Well, Joanne, have you been living in the area long?' Or 'Steve Sampler, that name sounds familiar – do you have relatives living in this area?'

Write it down: Keep a notepad and pen in handy places around the house, for example, next to every telephone, by the front door and in your car, so you can write down spur-of-the-moment ideas when they occur to you.

Keep thinking: Every day participate in some mental activity that requires your brain to remember, reason and react quickly. Do a crossword puzzle, play a word game, play chess, put away the calculator and do your own multiplication and division, read a book, debate politics with your partner, draw, paint, play a musical instrument, take a class at the local university or adult education centre, or write in a journal. Vegetating in front of the television may offer a good 30-minute break from a hectic day, but that shouldn't be your main form of recreation. The more you exercise your brain's ability to think, the better it will function.

Watch out for alcohol and other mind-numbing drugs. Most experts agree that a drink a day isn't health-threatening, but drinking too much can deaden your brain's ability to retain and recall information. Abuse of alcohol or recreational drugs can diminish your ability to absorb stimuli from the world around you and result in a limited ability to form new memories.

Most doctors agree that keeping your memory alive and well is simply a matter of following the basic advice offered throughout this section of the chapter: eat properly, exercise your body and exercise your mind. But you can use a few memory-enhancing quizzes, games and techniques to build your total recall.

Enhance Your Memory with These Methods

Most doctors agree that you don't need any formal mental gymnastics to keep your brain fit and functioning, but many people have found that certain techniques or activities have helped them hone their memory. The simple techniques offered here can give you a leg up in bolstering your ability to learn and recall new information.

Imagine this scenario: you're getting ready for work in the morning, and one of those morning news television programmes is chattering away in the background. You hear one of the announcers mention a product development that gives you an idea for one of the projects your team is involved in at work. You tell yourself you're going to research the product further once you get to the office and can discuss your ideas with your team. But by the time you're backing your car out of the drive, you've put the whole thing out of your mind. When you get to work, you have a sense that there's something you were going to do, but...

Events, ideas and information that pass into the hippocampus will pass straight on out again, unless you do something to set them down – by associating them with other memory that is already safely stored and ready for retrieval. The more associations the memory is tied to, the more likely you are to be able to store and retrieve it later. In psychology, this technique of associating new information with a range of memories for stronger recall is called elaborative encoding. It takes place in your frontal lobes – an area of your brain that always can use a good workout. Over the years, people have used a number of memory devices to aid this process:

Use the 'Roman Room': Ancient Romans used this practice to help them memorize long speeches, lists of objects, city names and so on. To try it, imagine a room. Then place around the room visual cues that remind you of items from your to-do list, shopping list or other types of information. A coat draped over a chair reminds you of the dry cleaning that needs to be picked up. A pair of skis leaning in the corner reminds you to call the travel agent about your plane tickets for your trip to Austria. Travel around the room in your mind, and make a mental note of sensory cues given off by the items – the colours, sounds and smells of the items, how they coexist with each other in the room, and any reaction they evoke in you. Make the images as vivid and compelling as possible. The room should continue to exist in your mind as a real place, with each of its furnishings a reminder of the things, people or events you want to lock in your memory.

Go into training for long-term lockdown: When you have stored information in your long-term memory – not just until you leave work or get through tomorrow's meeting – put your memory technique into a training programme. Review the information you need to remember at least three times a day for the next three to five days. At the end of your training programme, you should have the information safely in the vault.

Most of all, remember to work hard at preserving and building your cognitive functions, but try to enjoy the ride. After all, if you're worried about your memory, you probably aren't too far gone to get your ability to store and recall new information back up to speed.

CHAPTER 20

Keeping a Menopause Journal

A menopause journal can be an important tool for both you and your doctor. By chronicling your experiences, you create a clear vision of the physical and emotional changes you've experienced, to help you understand where you've been – and perhaps, where you're going – as you move into the next chapter of your life.

Why Should You Keep a Journal?

The perimenopause marks the beginning of another important phase of your life. And keeping a record of your evolution and the milestones you pass along the way can have important benefits for your body and mind.

Writing is good therapy, even for chronic illnesses. In an article published in 1999 in the *Journal of the American Medical Association*, doctors reported that writing about the experience of suffering from asthma and arthritis had a 'surprisingly beneficial effect on symptom reports, well-being and health care' for the individuals who recorded their experiences.

Your Journal as a Medical Record

A menopause journal serves a more serious purpose, but in much the same way. You keep a menopause journal to record the physical and emotional symptoms you experience each day as you move towards and through the menopause. Part of your journal will be a medical record, where you list physical observations, such as migraine headaches, irregular periods, sleepless nights, changes in your weight and so on. This same calendar should include your menstrual periods, so that if an association exists, you or your doctor will be able to notice. You aren't just keeping a record of your symptoms, but their severity, frequency and recurrence, so you can spot any patterns that occur.

Your doctors will benefit greatly from the information you've recorded in your menopause journal. They can use the information to gain a fuller picture of the way your symptoms are evolving and to gauge your response to medications and other treatment options you're exploring. If certain symptoms occur in tandem or in a specific sequence each month, especially in conjunction with your periods or with a lack of menstrual bleeding, that information may help your doctors better understand the specific triggering mechanism that prompts them.

Your Journal as a Personal Record

You also can use your journal to record your emotional symptoms and responses to the process of passing through the perimenopause and menopause. The very act of writing down your thoughts and feelings is a powerful tool for understanding them. Your journal gives you a much closer look at who you are, who you're becoming, what you most fear and what your hopes for the future entail. And the accurate record of the progress and patterns of your symptoms over the months in your journal actually can help you manage your reactions to some menopausal symptoms and expand your understanding of the process.

For example, your journal may record anxiety attacks, and in time you realize that those that wake you up at three AM and cost you hours of sleepless worry occur most often between the 10th and 14th days of your cycle. This understanding may enable you to say to yourself, 'This panic I'm feeling is a chemical response to hormonal fluctuations, not a true reaction to impending disaster.' With that, you may be able to do your deep breathing exercises, calm your mind and get back to sleep more quickly and surely.

tips

Continue your journal after the doctor prescribes any medical or hormonal therapy, or if you add an over-the-counter supplement to your routine, so that you can gauge any positive result or side effects over a period of time.

If you suffer from stress, just writing in your journal may give you a means for lessening the effects of this health-eroding condition. By writing about your stress – events that triggered the stress, your reactions and your thoughts about resolving the stress-inducing issues in your life – you give yourself a moment to stop the cycle of nervous tension, worry, anger and fear that add fuel and momentum to your stress.

Many women have noted that the perimenopause and menopause trigger feelings of introspection they haven't experienced before. If you find yourself thinking about your past, recollecting family holidays, relatives you haven't seen for years or your old boyfriends, write it down! These thoughts and ideas are important to you at this moment, or they wouldn't be occupying your mind. Making a record of them helps you take a broader look at exactly what about these past events may be saying to you now. Just remember to keep separate medical and personal journals, or transfer information from one journal into the symptom diary or calendar that you plan to take with you to your appointments.

Deciding What You Want Your Journal to Be

You can keep your menopause journal in any of a number of different forms and formats. Your journal can be as formal or informal as you choose it to be – you may write in a small, spiral-bound notebook; an unlined composition book; or one of the many leather or clothbound book-length journals for sale in most bookshops today. If you're a dedicated computer user, you may prefer to use any of the many journal-writing software programs, or you may prefer to write in a word-processing program and create your own journal organization. Your choices will be determined by when – and how – you use your menopause journal.

If you walk into a large bookshop or stationers today, you'll find a large selection of blank journals, beautifully bound and just waiting for your thoughts. Although you want to make sure that you'll enjoy keeping your journal (so you'll be more inclined to write in it on a regular basis), don't choose a journal format based on its cover appeal. You need a journal that will fit your lifestyle, your writing style and your habits.

That leather-bound, vellum-leafed book-style journal may make you feel like Jane Austen when you hold it in your hand, but how easy is it to write in? Will it lie open on the desk? Is it easy to balance on your knees? Are the pages too narrow to accommodate more than three words in your open, freehand scrawl? That journalling software may do everything but write your entries for you, but do you find that you're most inspired to write in your journal when you're away from your computer? Are the program's features too difficult to use or in the way for the type of writing you prefer to do?

Your menopause journal will be a very personal document, so only you can decide what shape and form it should be. Are you most comfortable writing by hand or with a keyboard? If you plan to use a computer, you need to be sure that yours is located in an area where you're comfortable relaxing and writing. If your computer is shared with other members of the family, you may prefer to set up some sort of password protection so that you can write what you choose to write without worrying about family members' reactions.

Taking a hard-copy journal away from home always leaves open the possibility that it will be lost or stolen. Travellers may want to keep a separate travel journal and transfer the information to a main journal when they return home. Always make back-up copies of electronic journals to prevent a loss due to hard disk failure or other computer-related mishaps.

Journal-writing software can help your organize, sort and search your entries to track recurrent physical and emotional issues over a period of time. If you plan to keep a hand-written journal, you'll want to find one that's the right size and shape for the types of records you want to keep. You may not want a week-at-a-glance-type layout, for example, if you want to do free writing, in which you may need ample space to write about your day. If you plan to keep numerous health records – headaches, menstrual cycle notes, diet information and so on – you may prefer some sort of lined pages that will help you neatly organize the information for fast reference.

Important Medical Information to Note

What kind of medical information and records do you want to maintain in your journal? In Chapter 3, we discussed the types of symptoms your doctor may want you to record in a monthly symptom diary. Most such records include a list, by the day of your menstrual cycle, of symptoms experienced and the severity of those symptoms (usually noted as mild, moderate or severe). Some typical symptoms included in symptom diaries or calendars are mood swings, irritability, insomnia, weight change, headache, increased appetite, fatigue, depression and forgetfulness. When you're preparing to begin your menopause journal, talk to your doctor to find out what symptoms he or she would most like for you to track over the next few months.

Although your menopause journal is much more than just this list of physical and emotional symptoms, those records are an important source of information for both you and your doctor, so choose them carefully. Here are some ideas:

Keep a diet journal: List the foods you eat, serving sizes and calorie counts if you're concerned about keeping track of the source of weight gain you may be experiencing or improving your nutrition. Many women have no idea how much they eat during the day or how well their diet conforms to the recommendations set forward by health experts. (See Chapter 13 for more information on those guidelines.) You may keep this as a separate journal, and you may keep it for a period of a few months only, depending upon your goals for the record. If you're trying to lose weight, you may want to list your weekly results with your diet record.

Keep an exercise journal: When you note the type of exercise you do each day, the length of time you exercise, number of repetitions and related information, you'll be able to check your progress and note any associations between your exercise, your symptoms, weight changes and overall feelings of well-being. This record can help encourage you to upgrade your exercise plan to keep it challenging and effective as your body's strength and endurance improve. The record also can give you an idea of which types of exercise seem to work best for you.

Track all cyclical symptoms: Many women experience cyclical symptoms as they move through the perimenopause. For example, hot flushes, migraine headaches or insomnia may occur at specific points in the menstrual cycles. Your symptom calendar will help you track these recurring symptoms. But you should also be certain to note days in which you have extraordinary feelings of calm, optimism or energy. Don't just be on high alert for negative days, but track the positive feelings as well. Your 'up' days may occur on a regular basis, and could provide you and your doctor with important information about hormone cycles, diet or other factors that contribute to them.

Note changes in medication or supplements: You don't need to begin each day's journal entry with a list of all of the vitamins and routine medications you've taken on that day; one entry in your journal should include that list for the record. But note any changes from your daily routine; add and remove medications as your prescriptions change or end, and note changes in the types or amounts of vitamin and mineral supplements you're taking. If you switch from brand-name prescriptions to generic, record that, too. If you forget to take any of your daily medications or supplements or run out of your supply temporarily, make sure that you note that – even if you have to go back later and add the information.

Checking your diet is also a helpful way to uncover connections between the foods you eat and menopause symptoms. You may discover that certain foods contribute to fatigue, hot flushes, headaches or insomnia. This is just one example of how your journal can offer important information about overall patterns of habits and symptoms that may occur during your menopause passage.

Finding Time to Write

Let's face it; your biggest challenge in writing a journal may not be choosing a format or deciding what kinds of information you most want to record. Beginning the habit of writing a journal is the most important part of the process, and it can be the most difficult as well. If you fail to keep your journal regularly, it loses much (but not all) of its value as a record of change; if you don't know where you've been, it's harder to understand where you may be going. Keeping a daily journal is a habit worth acquiring, however, so here are some ideas to help you in that effort:

Try to write at least once a day: If you can't bring yourself to note all of the items you think you should, at least write something. Like most worthwhile endeavours, journalling takes practice.

If time is a problem, 'automate' as much as possible: Find ways to create spreadsheets, checklists or other time-saving formats so that you can note items quickly that don't need a great deal of description. (You can pre-print daily diet lists, or devise your own shorthand system for noting symptoms.) If one form of journallng seems to be too time-consuming and you're tempted to stop, just try a different form. You're new at this, so you may not find your best method first go.

Begin by writing at the same time and in the same place every day: In time, you may choose to be freer in your approach to journalling, but when you're just getting started, setting a regular schedule may help you develop the habit.

Try timed practice: If you have a hard time writing about your feelings in your journal, try some timed exercises. Write whatever comes into your head for 10 to 20 minutes for three days in a row; you can describe the smell of a cup of coffee, your memories of your first kiss, a particularly nasty encounter you had at work that day, or reflections on your journey home. This kind of free writing can teach you to record your thoughts and open up to the writing process.

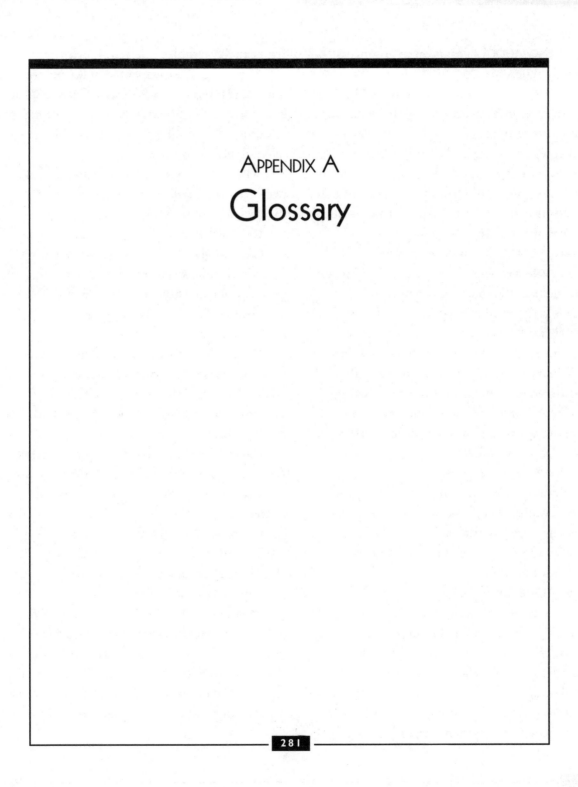

Appendix A
Glossary

AMENORRHOEA a cessation or absence of menstrual periods.

ANDROGENS male hormones normally produced in small quantities by the female ovaries and adrenal glands, with the greatest quantities occurring at the midpoint of a woman's menstrual cycle. Androgens are thought to promote a healthy sex drive and are sometimes prescribed as part of a full routine of hormone replacement therapy.

ANDROPAUSE *See* MALE MENOPAUSE.

ANGINA a squeezing, heaviness or tightness in your chest that happens when your heart muscle is deprived of oxygen.

ANTIOXIDANTS certain vitamins, including vitamins A, C, E and beta carotene, found in some brightly coloured fruits and vegetables, considered to be important tools in warding off heart disease and some cancers and in reducing age-related macular degeneration (age-related vision loss).

ATHEROSCLEROSIS a blood vessel condition that develops when the build-up of plaque on arterial walls narrows the arterial passage and thus limits the amount of blood that can flow through the arteries to nourish the heart, brain, kidneys and other organs.

BIOFEEDBACK a technique in which individuals are trained to monitor their breathing, heart rate and blood pressure (with the use of various instruments), then change their rate through relaxation techniques or visual imagery.

BIOFLAVONOIDS naturally occurring plant substances found in many brightly coloured fruits and vegetables, such as cherries, oranges, other citrus, grapes, leafy vegetables, red wine and some types of red clover. Bioflavonoids are being studied for the treatment of a number of conditions, including the control of bleeding, haemorrhoids and varicose veins.

BMI (BODY MASS INDEX) a measurement of a person's percentage of fat, determined by dividing a person's weight by their height.

CALCITONIN a hormone produced by the parathyroid gland to help regulate calcium levels in the bloodstream, and in so doing, protect bone density. Calcitonin is available in prescription form for the treatment of postmenopausal osteoporosis.

CARDIOVASCULAR DISEASE a term used to describe a variety of heart diseases, illnesses and events that affect the heart and circulatory system, including high blood pressure and coronary artery disease.

CERVICAL SMEAR a tissue sample taken (as a swab) during an internal vaginal exam to test for precancerous cell changes and cervical cancer.

CHEMOTHERAPY the use of potent medications to treat cancer, usually by affecting cells that are rapidly growing, such as the cancer cells themselves

CORONARY ARTERY DISEASE a common form of heart disease that results when the heart receives inadequate amounts of oxygen-rich blood through its arteries. This disease usually occurs when arteries become lined with heavy deposits of plaque – a substance made up of fat and calcium in a condition known as atherosclerosis.

DENDRITES the fine appendages at the ends of brain cells that transmit brain signals.

DEHYDROEPIANDROSTERONE (DHEA) an important hormone in the female body that decreases as a woman ages and declines dramatically after the menopause. DHEA is thought to combat memory and bone loss, and it may help to maintain breast and cardio-vascular health.

DEPRESSION an emotional disorder characterized by extreme or prolonged feelings of sadness, despair, guilt or hopelessness so debilitating that they affect one's normal quality of life and/or work performance.

DHEA *See* **DEHYDROEPIANDROSTERONE**.

ENDOMETRIAL CANCER cancer of the endometrium (womb or uterus).

ENDOMETRIAL HYPERPLASIA a precancerous condition of the endometrium that is typically diagnosed through a biopsy or sampling of the uterine lining, a procedure most doctors perform in their surgery.

ENDOMETRIUM the lining of the uterus.

ENDORPHINS naturally occurring substances released by the brain that resemble opiates, and are considered to be the brain chemicals that make you feel happy and content.

ESTRADIOL the main form of oestrogen produced by the ovaries, and the body's most efficient and potent oestrogen.

FIBROIDS benign growths of muscle cells that develop within or on the uterine wall.

FOLLICLE STIMULATING HORMONE (FSH) produced by the pituitary gland, promotes follicle development within the ovary, thus allowing certain eggs to mature and the follicle cells surrounding each egg to produce oestrogen in preparation for fertilization.

FSH *See* **FOLLICLE STIMULATING HORMONE**.

HDL CHOLESTEROL the high-density lipoprotein fraction of cholesterol ('good' cholesterol) that helps prevent heart disease by breaking up and carrying the low-density lipoprotein (LDL cholesterol) out of the bloodstream and into the liver for metabolism and evacuation in the faeces.

HEART PALPITATIONS the uncomfortable sensation that the heart is beating rapidly, out of sequence, too strenuously or in some other abnormal fashion.

HIPPOCAMPUS the part of the brain responsible for creating, storing and retrieving memory.

HORMONE REPLACEMENT THERAPY (HRT) therapy consisting of oestrogen or a combination of oestrogen and progestogen designed to replace the loss of these hormones in the menopause and thus combat the effects of this deficiency, including bone loss, vaginal dryness and hot flushes.

HOT FLUSHES hot flushes can be mild or severe, but in general, they involve a fast-spreading sensation of warmth through the face, neck and shoulders. Hot flushes are the result of fluctuating hormone levels, but their triggers, intensity and frequency vary from woman to woman. Hot flushes that occur during sleep are known as **NIGHT SWEATS**.

HRT *See* **HORMONE REPLACEMENT THERAPY**.

HYPERTENSION high blood pressure that occurs when arteries become too inflexible to allow an ample supply of blood to circulate, especially under periods of exertion or stress, thus causing excess pressure against arterial walls. Severe or ongoing high blood pressure can lead to strokes and other life-threatening conditions.

HYSTERECTOMY the surgical removal of the uterus that may or may not also be accompanied by the removal of the cervix and/or ovaries. If ovaries remain, the hysterectomy doesn't necessarily cause menopause, though menstrual bleeding ceases.

INDUCED MENOPAUSE a cessation of menstrual cycles that occurs when a woman has her ovaries surgically removed in a procedure called OOPHORECTOMY, or when a woman's ovaries cease to function prematurely as a result of medication, radiation, a lack of nutrition or excessive exercise. With treatment and intervention, some non-surgical types of induced menopause may be temporary. *See also* TEMPORARY MENOPAUSE.

INSOMNIA an inability to fall and/or remain asleep that occurs three or more nights a week.

ISOFLAVONES a type of plant oestrogen found in soya beans, red clover and (in much lower quantities) green tea, peas, pinto beans, lentils and other legumes, that may have benefits in treating some symptoms of the menopause.

LDL CHOLESTEROL Low-density lipoprotein cholesterol ('bad' cholesterol) is the fraction of total cholesterol that accumulates as fat deposits (plaques) on arterial walls.

LH. *See* LUTEINIZING HORMONE.

LUTEINIZING HORMONE (LH) a hormone produced by the pituitary gland, LH has multiple functions, one of which is prompting ovulation.

MALE MENOPAUSE known as ANDROPAUSE to the medical community, male menopause is associated with an age-related decrease in male hormone levels in men; symptoms can include lethargy, depression, mood swings, insomnia, hot flushes, irritability and decreased sexual desire and function.

MAMMOGRAM a low-dose X-ray of the breast used to screen for or examine lumps that may signify breast cancer.

MENARCHE the first menstrual period.

MENOPAUSE the permanent end of menstruation and fertility. *See also* NATURAL MENOPAUSE, INDUCED MENOPAUSE *and* TEMPORARY MENOPAUSE.

MIGRAINE HEADACHES intensely painful headaches thought to be associated with spasms in constricted blood vessels in the brain. Women who suffer migraines describe them as pounding headaches that can produce nausea, vomiting and a painful sensitivity to light, noise and smells.

NATURAL MENOPAUSE the cessation of all periods resulting from the halt of ovarian hormone production that is spontaneous and not the result of other physical or pathological conditions or treatments; natural menopause is diagnosed when a women has had 12 months of AMENORRHOEA.

NIGHT SWEATS *See* HOT FLUSHES.

NUTRACEUTICALS no legally determined or internationally accepted definition exists for this term, but in the marketplace it is used to describe foods or dietary supplements that claim to deliver some sort of medication or compound designed to offer a specific medical benefit.

OBESITY a condition of being more than 30 per cent over your ideal weight, or having a BODY MASS INDEX (BMI) of 25 or higher.

OESTROGEN a sex hormone produced by the ovaries, pituitary gland and (in small quantities) by body fat. During puberty, oestrogen stimulates the development of adult sex organs and the adult female breasts, hips and buttocks. Oestrogen helps to retain calcium in bones, regulates the balance of HDL and LDL CHOLESTEROL in the bloodstream and aids the maintenance of blood glucose level, memory functions and emotional balance.

OMEGA-3 FATTY ACIDS essential fatty acids found in fish, nuts, flaxseed, tofu and soya bean oils, that help nourish the hair and nails, and offer a number of benefits for cardiovascular health.

OOPHORECTOMY the surgical removal of one or both ovaries.

OSTEOPOROSIS a chronic disease in which a loss of bone mass results in porous, fragile bone that is prone to fracture. An age-related disease in the menopause, osteoporosis can manifest itself sooner in women who have risk factors.

OVULATION The release of a mature egg from a properly developed ovarian follicle.

PELVIC FLOOR EXERCISES a technique designed to strengthen the muscles of the pelvic floor to improve vaginal muscle tone, improve sexual response and limit involuntary urine release due to STRESS URINARY INCONTINENCE.

PERIMENOPAUSE the period of transition to natural menopause during which the body undergoes endocrinological and biological changes resulting from declining ovarian hormone production; symptoms can include irregular menstrual periods, hot flushes, vaginal dryness, insomnia and mood swings. The perimenopause can last up to six years (four years is average) and ends after 12 months of AMENORRHOEA.

PHYTOHORMONES natural substances found in some herbs and other plants that may help to regulate plant growth. Some types, referred to as phytoestrogens, can bind to the human body's oestrogen receptors and may act like an oestrogen or an anti-oestrogen on the body, depending upon their particular type and dosage.

PMDD *See* PREMENSTRUAL DYSPHORIC DISORDER.

PMS *See* PREMENSTRUAL SYNDROME.

POLYPS, UTERINE small, tag-shaped growths of uterine tissue, attached to the lining of the uterus. Polyps can cause irregular bleeding; doctors remove them to confirm there is no pre-cancerous change.

PREMENSTRUAL DYSPHORIC DISORDER (PMDD) a debilitating type of premenstrual syndrome that can include symptoms such as severe depression, anxiety, sleep disturbances and fatigue in addition to a wide range of physical disturbances. Although PREMENSTRUAL SYNDROME (PMS) and PMDD differ in severity, diagnosis and treatment, both seem to be linked to the way the body processes and responds to reproductive hormones and possibly serotonin.

PREMENSTRUAL SYNDROME (PMS) a condition occurring 10 to 14 days before the onset of menstrual bleeding and involving physical and emotional symptoms that include bloating, water retention, pelvic pressure or cramping, headaches or migraines, irritability, mood swings, difficulty concentrating and food cravings.

PROGESTERONE a female sex hormone produced in largest amounts during and after OVULATION that prepares the uterus for the implantation of a fertilized egg.

PROGESTOGEN a chemical name for various types of synthetic progesterone. Progestogen is used in HRT to balance the effects of oestrogen on the ENDOMETRIUM and prevent endometrial hyperplasia and cancer.

SELECTIVE ESTROGEN RECEPTOR MODULATORS (SERMS) a class of drugs used to help prevent bone loss. Raloxifene is one example of a SERM.

SERM See SELECTIVE ESTROGEN RECEPTOR MODULATORS.

STATINS cholesterol-lowering drugs.

STRESS URINARY INCONTINENCE the unpredictable and involuntary loss of urine caused by weakened sphincter muscles (the muscles that surround the urethra) and often triggered by an event such as a sneeze or cough.

TEMPORARY MENOPAUSE an interruption of the ovarian function that prevents the production of hormones that accompany the maturation and release of oocytes (eggs). Temporary menopause can follow chemical or radiation therapies or result from excessive exercise, weight loss or inadequate nutrition. See also INDUCED MENOPAUSE. When the contributing condition stops, ovulation and menstruation begin again.

TRIGLYCERIDES a type of fat found in the blood; other types of this fat include butter, margarine and vegetable oil. Triglyceride levels are checked in total fasting lipid-profiles (blood tests, sometimes called coronary panels, that check levels of HDL cholesterol, LDL cholesterol and triglycerides).

URETHRA the external opening in the bladder through which the body releases urine.

URGE INCONTINENCE involuntary bladder spasms that can be triggered by the sight, sound or even thought of water or urination; the sudden reflex need to urinate causes the spasm and an accompanying release of urine.

URINARY TRACT INFECTIONS (UTI) a bladder infection due to bacteria that typically has entered the bladder through the urethra through the process of intercourse, improper wiping techniques, poor hygiene, or other reasons.

UTI See URINARY TRACT INFECTIONS.

VAGINAL DRYNESS a condition characterized by the drying and shrinking of the vaginal lining. As the body's oestrogen production diminishes with menopause, the vagina produces fewer secretions, so the vaginal wall becomes less lubricated and flexible and more prone to tears and cracking.

VAGINITIS an infection due to bacteria, yeast or other pathogens, resulting in discomfort, itching and/or abnormal discharge.

VASOMOTOR SYMPTOMS hot flushes or night sweats that result from hormonal fluctuations in the menopause and perimenopause.

References
and Resources

Print and Online Articles, Journals, and Magazines

American Council on Exercise, 'Don't Deprive Yourself of the Rewards of Exercise', The American Council on Exercise Fit Facts, online, *www.acefitness.org*.

American Heart Association, 'Risk Factors and Coronary Heart Disease', American Heart Association Scientific Position, 26 November 2001.

Association of Reproductive Health Professionals, 'Mature Sexuality: Disorders of Desire and Alternative Approaches', ARHP Clinical Proceedings, electronic edition, December 1999, online, *www.arhp.org/clinical/cp12-99/cp12992.htm*

Bakos, Susan Crain, 'From Lib to Libido: How Women Are Reinventing Sex for Grownups', *Modern Maturity Magazine*, Sept/Oct 1999.

Brzezinski, Amnon, et al, 'Short-Term Effects of Phytoestrogen-Rich Diet on Postmenopausal Women', *Menopause: The Journal of the North American Menopause Society* 4, no. 2 (1997): 89–94.

Carandang, Jennifer, et al, 'Recognizing and Managing Depression in Women throughout the Stages of Life', *Cleveland Clinic Journal of Medicine*, 67, no. 5 (2000): 329–338.

Carpenter, Siri, 'Does Estrogen Protect Memory?', *Monitor on Psychology* 32, no. 1 (2001).

'Estrogen Lifts Mood in the Perimenopause', Women's Health Weekly News, reprinted in *Health & Sexuality*, Winter 2001.

Fisher, Linda. AARP/Modern Maturity Sexual Survey conducted by NFO Research, Inc., Washington, DC: AARP, 1999.

Guthrie, Janet R. and Lorraine Dennerstreing, 'Weight Gain, Somatic Symptoms, and the Menopause', *Menopausal Medicine* 9, no. 3 (2001).

'Health for Life', a special issue of *Newsweek* magazine, Fall/Winter 2001.

Holman, Marcia, 'Managing the Lesser-Known Effects of Estrogen Loss', MedscapeHealth, online, *www.health.medscape.com*.

Jacobs Institute of Women's Health Expert Panel on Menopause Counseling, 'Guidelines for Counseling Women on the Management of Menopause', Jacobs Institute of Women's Health, online, *www.jiwh.org*.

Kahn, David A., et al, 'Depression during the Transition to Menopause: A Guide for Patients and Families', in *Expert Consensus Guideline Series, A Postgraduate Medicine Special Report*, New York: The McGraw-Hill Companies, Inc., 2001.

Krauss, Ronald M., 'Diet and Cardioprotection: Sorting Fact From Fiction', *Menopause Management* 11, no. 1 (2002).

Kurtzweil, Paula, 'Lessening the Pressure: Array of Drugs Tames Hypertension', *FDA Consumer Magazine*, July–August 1999.

Mayo Foundation for Medical Education and Research, 'Headline Watch: New Evidence of ERT Risks', online, *www.MayoClinic.com*, 23 March 2001.

McNagny, Sally E., et al, 'Personal Use of Postmenopausal Hormone Replacement Therapy by Women Physicians in the United States', *Annals of Internal Medicine* 127 (1997): 1093–1096.

'Menopause', on The Alternative Medicine Channel, a member of HealthCommunities.com, online, *www.alternativemedicinechannel.com*.

Menopause Guidebook, Cleveland, OH: North American Menopause Society, 2001.

Murphy, Penelope, ed. *The American College of Obstetricians and Gynecologists Guide to Managing Menopause*. Washington, D.C.: ACOG, 2001.

Newton, K. M., et al, 'Women's Beliefs and Decisions About Hormone Replacement Therapy', *Journal of Women's Health* 6 (1997): 459–65.

'Physical Activity and Health: A Report of the Surgeon General', Center for Disease Control online fact sheet, *www.cdc.gov*.

'The Role of Isoflavones in Menopausal Health', Consensus Opinion of the North American Menopause Society. *Menopause: The Journal of the North American Menopause Society* 7, no. 4 (2000): 214–229.

Ryan-Haddad, Ann and Nasrin Piri, 'What Options Exist for Postmenopausal Breast Cancer Survivors with Hot Flashes?' *U.S. Pharmacist* 24, no. 9 (1999).

Scheiber, Michael D., et al, 'Dietary Inclusion of Whole Soy Foods Results in Significant Reductions in Clinical Risk Factors for Osteoporosis and Cardiovascular Disease in Normal Postmenopausal Women', *Menopause: The Journal of the North American Menopause Society* 8, no. 5 (2001): 384–392.

Smyth, J., et al, 'Effects of Writing about Stressful Experiences on Symptom Reduction in Patients with Asthma or Rheumatoid Arthritis', *Journal of the American Medical Association* 281 (1999): 1304–1309.

'Stealing Time', notes on the film by John Rubin and Ann Tarrant, PBS Online, *www.PBS.org*.

Still, Christopher D., 'Health Benefits of Modest Weight Loss', Healthology Press, online, *www.ABCNews.com*.

Takanishi, Gayle C., 'Drug Therapies for Hot Flashes in Breast Cancer Survivors', *Women's Health in Primary Care* 3, no. 11 (2000).

'Therapeutic Options During Perimenopause and Beyond', Section G of the Menopause Core Curriculum Study Guide, presented by the North American Menopause Society.

'Too Hot to Handle: Sex and Women over Fifty', in *Vitality: Health and Wellness for Midlife and Beyond*, online, *www.menopausehealth.com*.

Weinstein, Sheryl, 'New Attitudes Towards Menopause', *FDA Consumer Magazine*, March 1997 (revised February 1998).

'What Is Perimenopause?' on Menopause Online, *www.menopause-online.com*.

Wyon, Y., et al., 'Effects of Acupuncture on Climacteric Vasomotor Symptoms, Quality of Life, and Urinary Excretion of Neuropeptides among Postmenopausal Women', *Menopause: The Journal of the North American Menopause Society* 2, no. 1 (1950): 3–12.

Other Books on Menopause and Women's Health

Dooley, Michael and Stacey, Sarah, *Your Change, Your Choice: The Integrated Approach to Looking and Feeling Good Through the Menopause – And Beyond* (Hodder Mobius 2004)

Glenville, Marilyn, *Eat Your Way Through the Menopause* (Kyle Cathie 2002)

Glenville, Marilyn, *Natural Choices for Menopause: Safe, Effective Alternatives to Hormone Replacement Therapy* (St Martin's Press 1999)

Kenton, Leslie, *Passage to Power: Natural Menopause Revolution* (Vermilion 1998)

Lee, John R., *Premenopause: What Your Doctor May Not Tell You* (Little, Brown 1999)

Lee, John R. and Hopkins, Virginia, *What Your Doctor May Not Tell You About Menopause: Breakthrough Book on Natural Progesterone* (Little, Brown 1996)

Murray, Jenni, *Is It Me or Is It Hot in Here?: A Modern Woman's Guide to the Menopause* (Vermilion 2003)

Northrup, Christiane, *The Wisdom of Menopause* (Piatkus Books 2001)

Petras, Kathryn, *The Premature Menopause Book: When the 'Change of Life' Comes Too Early* (Quill 1999)

Stoppard, Miriam, Menopause: *The Complete Guide to Maintaining Health and Well-being and Managing Your Life* (Dorling Kindersley 2001)

Waterhouse, Debra, *Menopause Without Weight Gain: The Five-Step Solution to Challenge Your Changing Hormones* (HarperCollins 1999)

Weed, Susan, S., *New Menopausal Years: The Wise Woman Way* (Ash Tree 2002)

Professional Organizations and Informational Resources

British Menopause Society
4–6 Eton Place
Marlow
Buckinghamshire SL7 2QA
Tel: 01628 890199
www.the-bms.org

Royal College of Obstetricians and Gynaecologists
27 Sussex Place
Regent's Park
London NW1 4RG
Tel: 020 7772 6200
www.rcog.org.uk

NHS Direct
www.nhsdirect.nhs.uk
Tel: 0845 46 47

The National Osteoporosis Society (NOS)
Camerton, Bath BA2 0PJ
Tel helpline: 0845 4500 230
www.nos.org.uk

British Nutrition Foundation
High Holborn House
52–54 High Holborn
London WC1V 6RQ
Tel: 020 7404 6504
www.nutrition.org.uk

Diabetes UK
10 Parkway
London NW1 7AA
Tel helpline: 0845 120 2960
www.diabetes.org.uk

British Heart Foundation
14 Fitzhardinge Street
London W1H 6DH
Tel: 020 7935 0185
Heart information line: 0845 070 8070
www.bhf.org.uk

Cancer Research UK
PO Box 123
Lincoln's Inn Fields
London WC2A 3PX
Tel: 020 7009 8820
www.cancerresearchuk.org

Cancer BACUP
3 Bath Place
Rivington Street
London EC2A 3JR
Freephone helpline: 0808 800 1234
www.cancerbacup.org.uk

The Continence Foundation
307 Hatton Square
16 Baldwins Gardens
London EC1N 7RJ, UK.
Tel helpline: 0845 345 0165
www.continence-foundation.org.uk

Index